S.A.F. SIMPLIFIED
Self Awareness Formulas

From the research and writings of Joseph R. Scogna, Jr.

Kathy M. Scogna, editor

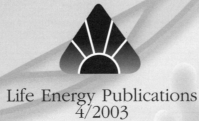

Life Energy Publications
4/2003

Acknowledgments: Special thanks to Nicholas T. Scogna for his painting of "The Sun: Key 19" which graces the cover of this book, and to Jezra Lickter for designing the CD-ROM, and giving us a presence on the web – www.scogna.com. Thanks to Joshua Lickter and Kalli Scogna for their typing, and Jason Scogna for being here. Each one has offered me love and support for which I am most grateful.

Thanks also to Jan Adams for her clarity and guidance, and to Jan and Kim and Bill at the Reading Eagle Press for helping to pull it all together.

This book contains portions of *The Secret of SAF, Life Force Discovery Program* and *The Science of SAF*, and is being presented so that another generation might comprehend the importance and share the vision of Joseph's research and works.

SAF Simplified - Self Awareness Formulas

Life Energy Publications – the only publisher of the complete and original works of Joseph R. Scogna, Jr.

Scogna, Kathy M., editor
  S.A.F. Simplified - Self Awareness Formulas

includes index
  1. self awareness 2. psychology   3. health
I. Joseph R. Scogna, Jr.   II. Kathy M. Scogna, editor III. title

ISBN: 0-9652292-5-4

Printed by Reading Eagle Press, Reading, Penna. USA

S.A.F. SIMPLIFIED
Self Awareness Formulas

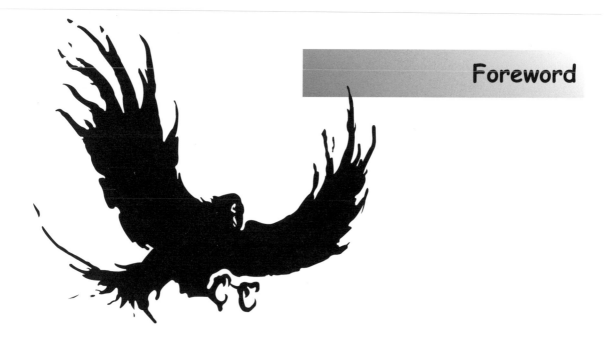

Foreword

For at least the last 5,000 years of recorded history, medicine and spirituality were aligned in natural philosophy. While many Asians followed the tenets of Lao Tzu who wrote down the ancient teachings into the *I Ching,* the Greeks followed the study of the humors, the progression a disease takes as experienced by symptomatology. In these natural philosophies, illness was not considered a specific disease but rather a collection of symptoms brought on by an imbalance. Once this imbalance was corrected, harmony would be restored. The purpose was to bring about balance.

With the invention of the microscope, the formerly invisible became visible and a new world opened up. A schism occurred in natural philosophy. Medicine/science took a sharp turn on the path to address only what was visible (1% of reality) leaving philosophy/spirituality to grapple with the invisible.

Our base of knowledge is greater today than in the past, but are we smarter than the ancients? Of the writings that remain it would appear we have lost something dynamic – our will to know ourselves as a composite of body, mind and spirit.

While the microscope has been justly heralded for its benefits to mankind, it has also led to our downfall as perceptual beings. No longer are we allowed to intuitively know and understand life or explore our spiritual selves.

Knowledge must now be <u>seen</u> for it to be true. And that duty of seeing and diagnosing has been relegated to the doctor and lab technician with the microscope. We lost our capacity to understand the invisible, which makes up 99% of existence. We became patients, patiently waiting for the doctor to give a title to our ailment and then to be bombarded with the latest coal tar-derived medicines. Never a word about balance. Anyone who even whispered the word "balance" was dismissed as a quack and driven out.

Joseph R. Scogna, Jr. was not one to accept the status quo. He was able to peer down the time track of humanity looking for the energetic solutions to the troubles of man, his symptoms, his imbalances. On this mental trek, Joseph took with him an understanding of cosmic and atomic energy and he applied this to the studies of the past, specifically symptomatology as found in homeopathy, the humors of the Greeks and the balance of the *I Ching*. He used philosophical reflection and various modern machines, including computers and infrared, to define the electroplasmic field around living beings, Life Energy, and to codify the metabolic connections of body, mind and spirit. He dismissed the word "patient," brought back the word "balance," and has given mankind a modern day natural philosophy that incorporates the visible and the invisible.

SAF, the Self Awareness Formulas, is Joseph Scogna's published research into symptomatology and these metabolic connections of body, mind and spirit. In *SAF Simplified*, the reader is encouraged to discover his or her own awareness level and then learn to increase that level. For it is through self knowledge that we grow. It is through self awareness that we can bring about balance in our lives. This balance and harmony in our own lives will create a ripple that will affect all mankind.

—Kathy M. Scogna
May, 2003

Table of Contents

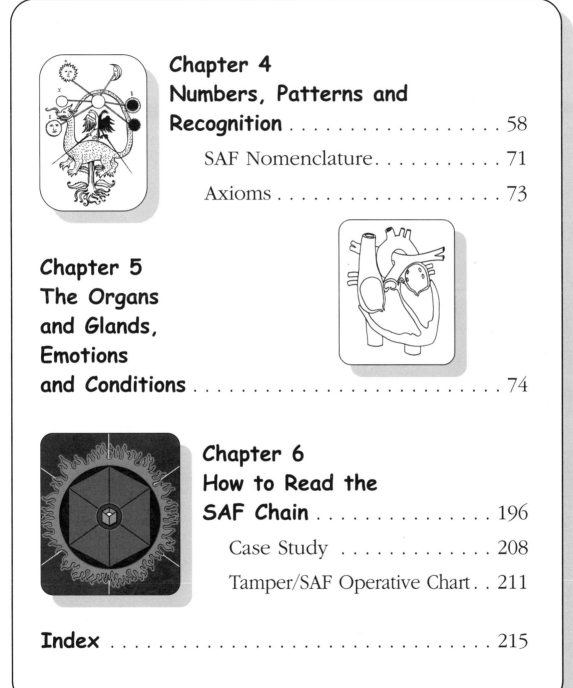

A Quick Tour,
or How to use this Book and CD-ROM

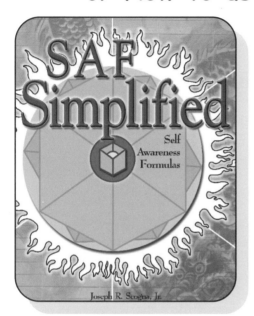

This book and CD-ROM have been designed to help you discover for yourself what the Self Awareness Formulas called S.A.F. have to offer. SAF is a practical application of the theories and writings of Joseph R. Scogna Jr., considered by many to be a pioneer in his field.

Your health and well being have always been your responsibility. But what do you do if you can't see the cause of your problems? Now, with these Self Awareness Formulas, there is a method for you to understand yourself and your loved ones. You can now discover what your symptoms mean and most importantly, you'll learn how to dissolve old patterns and make positive changes in your life. (In SAF, we like to say you'll learn to face your dragons.) By utilizing the specific methods and formulas available with SAF each of us can overcome emotional traumatic stumbling blocks and greatly enhance our own mental telepathic powers.

Thousands have studied the SAF method of self awareness through practitioners' offices. It is now available to the general public in an easy to understand format – SAF SIMPLIFIED. People just like you have regained their self determinism regarding their health, their life and their business.

How is this possible?

How can one method cover so much territory?

SAF will give you the opportunity to see your problems in a new light, and then something magical will happen. A spark of understanding occurs, energy is released, the path becomes clear.

Is your situation an emotional issue of long duration?

Business trouble?

Recurring behavior pattern?

Aches and pains of unknown cause?

In short, whatever problem areas you have can be addressed with self awareness and self knowledge. Throughout the book, you'll learn how the mind works, and how unresolved traumas from the past can influence you and your behavior in the present. You'll learn how and why this particular self awareness program – SAF – is so personal and so effective.

It is recommended that you read SAF SIMPLIFIED completely to get a working understanding of the theory behind SAF and why it works. Then, pop the CD-ROM into your computer, answer the questions on the SAF Stress – 120 Questionnaire, and you will receive your own SAF chain of numbers. Chapter 6 will give you a worksheet with step by step instructions on how to decipher your SAF chain. The CD-ROM is designed to run on both IBM and MAC computers.

It's easy! It's fun! But more importantly, it will change your life. You may use the CD-ROM as often as you wish to help yourself and your family gain greater awareness of the messages your symptoms are (and have been) trying to tell you.

You are now about to depart on an interesting journey, one of self-discovery and adventure.

"You cannot teach a man anything – you can only help him to find it within himself." —Galileo

The CD that was included with this book created a chain only. **Due to computer upgrades since 2003, it no longer worked.** To create an SAF chain to use with this book, please visit www.LifeEnergyResearch.com and complete the Stress-120 Questionnaire. This is a free service!

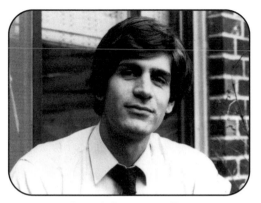

Joseph R. Scogna, Jr.

Chapter 1

SAF: A Light in the Darkness

In This Chapter

➤ Man versus superman
➤ Immunity
➤ What is self awareness?
➤ How can SAF connect sciences?
➤ Doesn't time heal all wounds?
➤ How can a past event haunt someone?
➤ How can numbers tell the way I feel?
➤ How does SAF work?

What is S.A.F.?

S.A.F. stands for Self Awareness Formulas. These formulas are actually from a collection of works written by Joseph R. Scogna, Jr. in the 1980s, which includes books, course materials, medical evaluations, questionnaires and computer programs.

Joseph was a brilliant researcher, who cross-connected physics, mathematics, nutrition, modern western medicine and ancient eastern philosophies to create what he called the science of SAF. It is truly the science for future man. Its purpose is to increase the awareness of every man, woman and child on many levels, always encompassing the body, the mind and the spirit. This is accomplished through symptom awareness, whether it is physical or emotional symptoms, business or family situation issues.

At the very first seminar on SAF in 1980, the people in attendance were absolutely floored by the information. Even Joseph, the inventor, was surprised. He was heard to say, "I didn't think it would do this, not this quickly!"

What did SAF do?

The first thing SAF did was to take the mystery out of symptoms. A simple question-naire was filled out and the answers were decoded. Much to the surprise of those in attendance, Joseph was then able to tell each person:

A – what conditions were manifesting in the present

B – what situations had occurred before the present day condition

C – based on mathematical probability, what conditions were likely to appear in the future.

SAF helped steer each person to the correct order in which he or she should proceed against the problems. For example, if one person had eight symptoms, the SAF pointed out the preferred order for addressing these.

SAF also prioritized what modalities should be used, such as vitamins, minerals, enzymes, glandular preparations, herbs, homeopathic remedies, exercise, diet, etc.

But probably the most exciting thing SAF did on that day was give the seminar atten-dees a tool to measure themselves against higher, more intelligent beings.

Man vs. Superman

Carl Jung preached a philosophy in the middle 20th-century that bespoke of the differ-ence between man and superman (he called superman "Übermensch" in his native tongue, German). In vogue at the time were various theories propounding the origina-tion of the human species, the most prominent being Darwinism. While Charles Darwin was touting how much human beings resembled monkeys and vice versa, Jung and others expounded on how much people were like God. Differences in human behavior were regularly compared to the actions of God and monkey alike.

When SAF appeared on the scene, it froze forever in a cryogenic display case the archaic foibles of these sciences, for SAF could cause a proper distinction between the man who was God-like and the man who behaved more like an ape.

A Scale to measure Progress

With Carl Jung's philosophy in mind, the SAF Scale of Unified Existence was written in order to measure progress. At the bottom is 0 as nonexistence (not death – death is about 2.5 on the scale) and at 1000 is Übermensch (superman or Unchained Spirit). We desperately try to move up the scale if we want to flourish or down if we want to suc-cumb. Of course, very few of us consciously want to be vaporized.

How do we move on this scale? How do we attain health and healing?
Seminars conducted by the founder of SAF with various groups netted these answers:

Medical Doctor: "Destroy all foreign organisms in the body with the healthy use of antibiotics."

Massage therapist: "Restore electromagnetic balance to the body, mind and spirit with daily massages."

Chiropractor: "Eliminate nerve blockage with spinal adjustments."

Naturopath: "Correct biochemistry with herbs and proper nutrition."

Spiritual person: "Eliminate negative thoughts through meditation and prayer."

Astrologer: "Observe proper astral cycles of behavior."

Taoist: "Pursue a middle course. Thus will you keep a healthy body and a healthy mind."

Shinto: "Foster a spirit that regards both good and evil as blessings, and the body spontaneously becomes healthy."

Macrobiotic: "Five parts grain, two parts vegetables - cook with a peaceful mind, eat with a spirit of gratitude."

Buddhist: "All living beings owe their present state of health to their own karma."

Nutritionist: "Organic whole foods, with supplements of enzymes, vitamins and minerals are essential for optimum functioning."

Many societies and groups were contacted for answers concerning the movement of a person away from annihilation and up the scale of existence toward Übermensch.

Who was right?

All were, and none were. The bottom line seemed to be that what works for some doesn't work for all. So people move from practice to practice, modality to modality, in a quest to attain the status of Übermensch. But how would we know we were Übermensch if we became one? Was there a common denominator?

Immunity

The word immunity has been spoken so many times by orthodox practitioners and in medical journals, could it be that SAF and orthodox medicine have something in common?

Yes. But those schooled in SAF wonder how a person can gain immunity by always making war and not peace. The very word antibiotic has a belligerent attitude. Anti (against) biotic (life) means to war on life. By taking antibiotics, we aren't building immunity we're making war. The war is against microorganisms, to be sure, but the microorganisms are bothering us because we're not immune (not at peace). So the orthodox theory says, "I'll fix those blankety-blank bugs. I'll incinerate them with my new squadron of erythromycin." The only problem is, after a good term of these skirmishes within the boundaries of the body, the patient looks and feels like a war zone during a major offensive.

As contrary as it may sound, immunity is gained by <u>making peace</u>. Super Immunity, the kind Übermensch possesses, is gained by a vast ability to make peace with all entities on earth. There are people who have ongoing wars with common substances such as chocolate, wheat, milk and corn to name a few. If a person nips at a piece of chocolate and falls over in anaphylactic shock, he certainly is a long way from 1000 on the Übermensch scale. He is more likely at 3.

Übermensch is in Total Harmony and Absolute Serenity with his environment. He has Total Immunity.

Is achieving Übermensch a pipe dream?

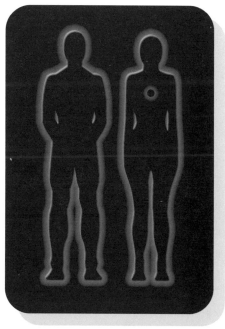

People reading this text are floating between 3 and 7 on the Übermensch scale. Their immunities are low. They have ongoing wars with the atmosphere, pollution, water, food, emotions and business.

Split these categories up into finer and finer parts and we have in front of us a tonnage of travail. For example, someone may be afraid of the dark; the dark wars on him. When it gets dark, the soldiers of emptiness invade his mind spaces and surround him. So, he needs to gain immunity (make peace) with the dark.

All manner of entity shape and form can make war on an individual. Some examples would be a dog, the face of an ex-lover, ice cream, the smell of wood (trees), a car, air-conditioning vapors, angry words, certain sounds, specific locations.

Übermensch is in Total Harmony and Absolute Serenity with the environment.

In other words, to have Total Immunity (on body, mind and spirit levels) there can be no fear, no stress and no anguish. Übermensch, with Total Immunity, has <u>no allergies</u>. If Übermensch were shot with a bullet, his body would just spit the lead out because Übermensch is immune to bullets. Not only is he immune to bullets, but he is immune to the hate and negative emotions that caused the bullet to be fired toward him in the first place.

Can Übermensch, or a slight facsimile of him, be had for humankind? SAF is where you will begin your journey of self discovery.

Is SAF a personality test?

No, it's not a psychological evaluation or an IQ test. SAF is not like anything you've ever seen before. It is a precise examination, and yet this is not a cookie-cutter solution, one size fits all. Because it was designed to cross-connect all sciences and philosophies, it employs various approaches, such as questionnaires, standard blood and urine tests, hair analysis, biofeedback data, infrared detection, and others.

Its title, Self Awareness Formulas, signifies that it is used to increase your awareness. . . about yourself.

What is self awareness?

These particular Self Awareness Formulas (SAF) will teach about the interconnections between the body, mind and spirit for the purpose of improving lives. Through self knowledge, we can learn to understand, experience and breakdown barriers in order to get to the next higher level of understanding. Greater self awareness allows us to integrate more knowledge, and as we continually move upscale, we can assume greater responsibility for the creation and sustenance of our own power and health.

Who would want to use SAF?

Because it is about increasing self awareness, the reasons for working with SAF are as varied as there are people on planet earth. SAF is for those who want to seize the day and make a difference in their life and the lives of their loved ones. For others, there may be traumas from long ago that are haunting and affecting them, or perhaps they are not satisfied with simply existing. Still others may have allergies to or ongoing wars with foods, people, alcohol and emotions.

People use SAF as a realigning tool to dissolve old behavior patterns, and to bring about resolution to situations that they want to change. If given the choice, we each have a trouble or two in our lives that we could do without. It might be a physical symptom, or an emotional issue, or a situation with our boss, spouse, children or parents.

But the fact is we DO have a choice. In fact, we make choices everyday. But somehow either we make the wrong choice and our life never improves, or the same old problem creeps up on us again and again. After awhile, we come to the conclusion that life is too complicated to understand fully.

Why is life so complicated sometimes?

The reason why things seem so complicated is because the answers for important questions remain unknown. We might think we have the solution but then it doesn't always hold true. Or something changes in our life and it seems we are right back where we started.

Can life be made simpler?

Yes – simplicity is the opposite of difficulty. It is accomplished by applying known information to any complex situation to make the complex situation more easily understood. This process is the most basic learning routine. For example, when a baby is born into the world, everything is foreign and complicated. However, by using a step-by-step process of association, the baby can ultimately learn about his environment. He uses the learning technique that has been handed down through the generations since the beginning of time. A child learns by experience.

This learning routine – experience – is based on the "feelings" of the individual. When something "feels good," then it is thought to be right. When something "feels bad" then it is believed to be wrong. An adult continues to learn by experience in this same way.

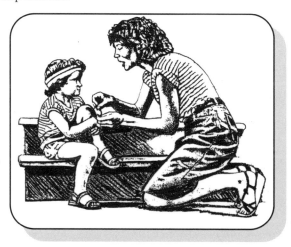

The term that is used for right feelings is called happiness. We all want to find ways to increase our quotient of happiness. Much happiness is called well being.

The word used for wrong feelings is sadness. A good deal of sadness is known as DISEASE.

We learn "good" from "bad" through experience.

What do you mean by disease?

In SAF, a disease is a complication too severe or too large to comprehend. It means that you have a problem, any kind of problem, that you can't solve. We use the word "insoluble" to denote a problem that can't be broken down into its finer parts. Your mechanism for breaking down your problem becomes inhibited and therefore causes distress or discomfort. This type of distress is the SAF definition of disease, or dis-ease.

How does a person make himself feel better?

To feel better is as simple as solving a problem. The word problem means a puzzling or difficult circumstance; it's synonymous with heaviness and pressure. It implies the notion of impenetrable mass.

To solve a problem, we must dissolve it. We do this primarily by breaking down the problem into smaller bits so it is easier to understand. It is difficult for us to solve a great problem without first taking it apart. Once the problem is dissected, it can be understood more easily.

For example, if you were to attend a university to study physics, chemistry or medicine, you couldn't understand all the ramifications of these sciences in a single one-hour long class. You must become a student and analyze these bodies of knowledge one piece at a time. You must learn the language of the subject; you must feel your way through the various courses until you know it from the inside out. Anyone who has ever said he could learn a whole science by just glancing at one textbook is fooling himself. It takes concentration and effort, and necessitates splitting the subject into smaller pieces.

When we have a problem, we must provide remedies to solve the problem and, of course, the remedy must match the problem.

How do remedies really work?

The right remedy always solves the problem. We can find examples with our own bodies to prove this. For example, when we're hungry, we are presented with the problem of having a particular uncomfortable sensation in our stomachs and a gradual loss of energy. The remedy of course would be to provide our body with food.

For another view, let's say that a person cut himself. The immediate problem would be the body signaling that there is a tear in the skin, with the usual symptoms of bleeding, pain and swelling. If the person wanted to solve this problem, then he would provide a clamp or Band-Aid that would close up the cut, or perhaps he would need to be stitched.

In another example, if you miss another person very badly, then your body will receive signals through your mind and viewpoint by providing an aching feeling in the heart. Each of us has our own way of signaling ourselves when we miss someone, but generally there is a feeling of disconnection. The remedy for this particular problem is to supply the missing person and relieve the pain of separation.

In some cases, however, we miss someone who cannot be replaced and therefore a very specific remedy to adjust our viewpoint is needed.

The proof as to whether or not this program has been successful would be the symp-

> *SAF is not medical diagnosis. Physical diseases have underlying emotional causes – some may be very deep indeed. It is this aspect of the human being that we address in the science of SAF."*   —*Joseph R. Scogna, Jr.*

toms that alerted us about the problem in the first place. Are the symptoms of disconnection or aching heart still present?

When the symptoms are removed, we feel better, and when we feel better we feel "right" about our existence.

Can anyone feel better and stay better?

Theoretically, if symptoms were taken away, we would always feel good. We could logically conclude that the reason for our disaffection for disease is the fact that we must bear symptoms. But we can't simply take symptoms away and not eliminate their causes, because the symptoms would just keep reappearing.

Almost all disease and physical ailments are caused by mental or spiritual distress. The answer to getting better and staying better is to consistently upgrade our awareness of the causes and effects of mental, physical and spiritual symptoms. So, symptom awareness is crucial.

Man, since the beginning of time, has tried to observe his relationship with the environment to learn more about himself through many studies, such as philosophy, chemistry, biology, physics, medicine, religion and the like. But the most important subject of all is the study of human beings.

What is a human being?

In the simplest definition of a human being, we could say that he or she is composed of body, mind and spirit. Each of these divisions, if you will, has its own separate science and awareness. Today, medical science and physiology are attempting to increase their know-how and awareness of the body and its processes; psychology and related sciences of the mind are attempting to accumulate more information on mental abilities; and religion and spirituality have always had the spirit in its bailiwick.

> *Man is a composite of spirit, mind and body.*

Is there a science that deals with the whole person – body, mind and spirit?

Yes. SAF is a universal tool for understanding the connections of body, mind and spirit. It's a method that includes and uses all sciences. *The Secret of SAF: The Self Awareness Formulas of Joseph R. Scogna, Jr.* is an in-depth study of this unique approach to health and well being. In addition, there are other books on complementary areas of study, such as *The Promethion, The Threat of the Poison Reign* and others that utilize the SAF interface.

How does SAF use all sciences?

SAF deals with the interrelationships of all sciences that affect the human person and its environment. In short, the science of SAF can be applied to any body of knowledge to measure it. In *The Secret of SAF* mentioned above, sixty-four of the dichotomies of these bodies of knowledge are explained as they relate to the human being.

How can SAF connect sciences?

SAF can connect sciences because it is based on the most fundamental knowledge there is – mathematics.

Do I have to know a lot of math to use SAF?

No, there are no tabulations necessary with this book as it contains a CD-ROM. There is no new math or old math for that matter.

Then how is mathematics used in SAF?

In our everyday life, we use numbers to measure the magnitude and quantity of objects, places and things. Any science that employs quantities or qualities must have numbers for its basic measurement. You will find that all sciences and all conditions must yield to numbers. Galileo wrote a true statement: the story of the entire universe was written in the language of mathematics. A mathematical matrix is an integral part of SAF and so it is able to connect all sciences. Numbers comprise the language of SAF.

Then what is a number?

A number is a symbol that represents a quantity or quality. A number has no feelings until it is assigned feelings, no energy until it is endowed with energy. SAF assigns qualities such as feelings, emotions and energy to numbers.

How can numbers tell the way a human being feels?

The numbers 1-24 are used in the science of SAF. Let me give an example of how we use the number 6. In the assignment of the organs and glands of the human body number 6 is assigned to the liver. In the breakdown of emotions, the number 6 is dubbed sadness, while the condition given for number 6 is transmutation. In each particular study listed with SAF programming (880 in all), there is a separate meaning for the number 6. This is not a statement to impress anyone with the enormity of the science of SAF, but merely to show that a number can mean different things in various bodies of knowledge.

SAF utilizes a chain of numbers (2-1-4-7) to represent the organ and gland complex (heart-thymus-stomach-lungs) or the emotions (love-aggression-happiness-monotony).

In this book we will use four meanings for each number.

With SAF methods, these number designations and their meanings are then prioritized. They can be put into a sequence of importance that has meaning for that particular person and that person alone. The only true meaning of existence comes in the way of a sequence.

What do you mean by a sequence?

A sequence is a number of items following one another, a progression. In SAF we follow the chain link of energy of which everything is made, and we create sequences of numbers. Here on planet earth, man has learned to live with his sequences and understand them to a certain extent. Philosophers and scientists who understand many sequences of energy have led the population out of their misunderstandings about life; these were learned men such as Socrates, Plato, Lao Tzu, Hippocrates and Einstein to name but a few.

Each human being must learn the basic sequences of existence in order to survive. Any event that occurs on earth must precede or succeed another event, and we call this action TIME.

The examples of time are many. Everything must take time, and for time, there are sequences.

For example, the corn on the cob that was served at dinner was produced by a sequence of events through time. The corn came from a seed and that seed came from another corncob. There is a complete series of events that take place in order to produce an ear of corn. Each ear of corn must have a birth, then grow and mature into a ripened state, and then eventually decay until its final death or demise. We take the corn in its ripened state and eat it for nourishment. This sustenance helps us create sequences of energy in our own bodies.

In another example of a sequence, a human being is born and grows to an age at which he or she is fit to behave as a mature adult. Eventually we begin to grow older, decay and then reach a point in our lives when we must face the finish of our existence as a human being – death. Again, this is a sequence of time. It is a succession of energy; it is a chain link of past and present events upon which we can speculate about the future.

As we grow older, we can look back on our earlier lives and see our own sequences. If we are in good shape and have good recall, the emotional cycles and patterns of our behavior are apparent.

It is the tracks of time that control human beings, and SAF tracks time. We create sequences of numbers to do this.

But how can SAF tell how we feel in time?

SAF tracks time and intensity. Remember that a person must assign some significance to an event in this time sequence and assign it some feelings. The intensity for this significance comes from the individual. For example, if you wanted to go to the store to have an ice cream cone, then you may assign significance to this event as being pleas-

Incident 1

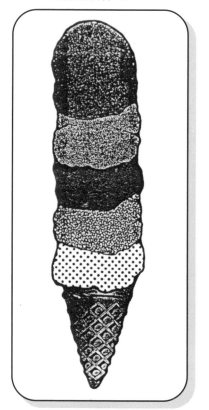

Incident 2

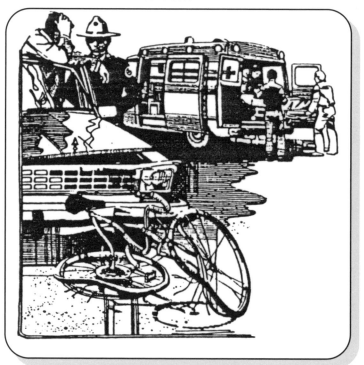

At left: an enticing ice cream cone. Above: an unhappy car accident.

ant. However, if one day on the way back from the ice cream store, you are in a car accident, then you may award a very different kind of significance to this event. You may term this event unpleasant, and in unpleasant circumstances, we perceive intensity, pressure and stress.

But once that sequence is over, we should get better, right? Doesn't time heal all wounds?

Yes it is true to a certain extent. We do have self-regeneration mechanisms that can heal us, but the <u>intensity</u> of the event and the <u>strength</u> of the regeneration capabilities are the real factors, not time. If we were weak to begin with, we may never get over the trauma of the accident. Because we are unique individuals, different people recover from similar events in differing lengths of time.

How can a past event haunt a person? Why can't we just blot a trauma out of our memories?

Let's look at the two events again, pleasant and unpleasant. Your body and mind have the ability to record everything so you can remember it for future reference. This is part of the learning process. In the unpleasant event, the ice cream cone was retrieved (bringing pleasure) but you had to pay for it with some pressure and stress (the accident).

The following graph shows the differences in energy as they are recorded in the body. In the pleasant event, the energy is light, airy and without stress. In the unpleasant event, the energy is com-

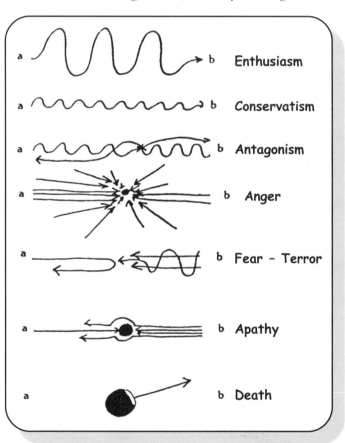

The differences of energy as recorded in the body. The eating of the ice cream cone, incident #1, would fall on the above graph at the Enthusiasm State, light, airy, and without stress. The accident, on the other hand, incident #2, would probably fall between anger and death since it is compressed, mean and stressed.

pressed, angry, mean and stressed. It is power-packed with energy and worse – the images have become so ensnarled in the pressure that the individual cannot tell one event or sequence of events from the other. Incident #1, the ice cream cone adventure, can be easily recalled. Incident #2 may not be remembered at all. The events could be cloudy and confused in the mind of the person.

In the case of a car accident, even a fender-bender, people often don't remember what led up to the accident or what immediately followed, even though they were said to be fully conscious.

Remember that there are certain amounts of intensity, stress and pressure associated with trauma.

How can this kind of pressure affect my health?

Your well being depends on your view of life. If your mind is clouded by negative emotions such as hate, anger, fear, and mental troubles, these hostile feelings will eventually affect you physically as well.

How can a negative emotion affect physical well being?

Remember that we learn by experience. Emotions are made of energy; they are the experience of life in the environment. Emotions are mental experiences, which have biochemical (physical) significance and tell your body how to be, how to feel.

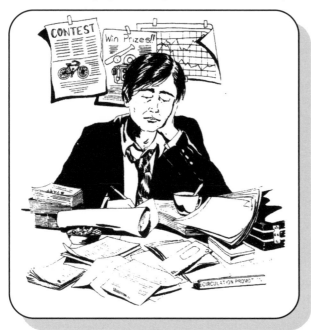

A person's well being depends on his or her view of life. If the mind is clouded by negative emotions, then the physical state will suffer.

So, is all emotion bad?

No. Emotion is something that occurs in a healthy human being. It is something that when used for the proper circumstances, provides pleasure and enjoyment in life in a positive way. The word "emotion" means expressed or electrified motion.

Remember the ice cream cone sequence and how the mental pictures became ensnarled and confused? It is the impact and intensity of experience that confused the expression of motion – emotion – in the body.

Have you ever hear someone say, "I don't know how to feel?" It means the person's memory banks and experiences are so befuddled and balled up that any old feeling may come squirting out at the wrong time.

For example, the ice cream cone accident may present the following confusion of emotion (reminders):

Ice cream	fun and tasty
Driving	exhilaration
Ice and snow	pretty but be careful
Cold and wet	uncomfortable
Slip on the ice	out of control
Metal hitting metal	impact, unconsciousness, pain, anger, hurt and bewilderment
Ambulance	spinning lights, flashing lights, sirens
Hospital	scared and worried
Stitches	pain and confusion
Drugs	numb, confused, disoriented and vomiting

As you can see, there is a confusing disarray of emotions. Having all this under control in your mind and body is the ultimate secret weapon against confusion. After a car crash you may be able to write a best selling novel and become famous for it, but what if this event and others like it are lost inside your memory banks and never work their way out? What if this abnormal event cannot be controlled and therefore becomes confused in your normal processes of emotion?

In the science of SAF the traumas that exert their influence outside of your control are affectionately called "dragons." It is through an examination of these trauma/dragons that we can learn more and gain greater awareness about ourselves. We welcome dragons.

Down through the ages, dragons have been used by all cultures to represent the unseen and the unknown – definitely a force with which to be reckoned. These trauma/dragons can present themselves in a number of unwanted ways, such as becoming mixed up with your everyday feelings, causing you to react unreasonably and illogically.

This is what could happen:

Any reminder of the ice cream cone car accident in our sample can trigger a reaction. The key word here is <u>reminder:</u> it means to put into the conscious mind again.

Any reminder of the event, whether you are conscious of it or not, could start the whole chain sequence of emotions and patterns of that former event (car accident) occurring once again. This means that you will actually feel the same sensations and pains as you did when you were in the accident. These expressions of motion can all occur without control and on their own volition.

Now go back to the make believe "ice cream cone car accident" and find the list of confusing emotions. These are called the reminders. What are they? Remember that the mind has been squashed and one reminder is as good as the next.

The mention of "ice cream" stimulates the earlier "unhappy car accident" event; it presses on the consciousness without your consent, exerting its own control over you. You may be able to see only the ice cream cone but feel the rest of the now jumbled sequence.

Any one of the feelings or actions in the event can be a reminder.

Have you ever had a bad experience and then someone later asked you about the incident and you said, "Please. . . don't remind me"?

You could be out at a party enjoying yourself when a friend asks if you would like to have some ice cream. Your mind and body become confused and take the reminder "ice cream" to signify <u>an impending disaster or collision</u>. This is because the pleasure of eating ice cream had become mixed in with all the other negative experiences of the accident. So instead of feeling good, you now feel bad about the thought of ice cream, for no reason known to you.

These "bad feelings" occur to us all the time. They can be just fleeting thoughts, a flashback or they can flood in without an understanding of their origin. This is often the case with *déjà vu* experiences. They can have a tremendous and disruptive influence in your life.

Why does the person feel bad? The accident was in the past. It can't hurt him now, can it?

In our "ice cream cone car accident" the reminders could come without the person's conscious permission or even recognition. Here are some possible "ice cream cone accident" reminders:

> An ambulance speeding by
>
> The sound of a siren in the distance
>
> Having fun
>
> Someone being angry
>
> Something that tastes good

Notice that "having fun" could remind the individual of the "ice cream cone accident." The mind and the body are logical, but only when they are in good working order. Remember that we learn by our experiences, the automatic recording of these experiences, and in this case "having fun" and "car accident" are all jumbled together.

Remember the mind and body have been programmed to avoid pain and death at all costs. This is why human beings seek pleasure and avoid uncomfortable situations that involve pain.

The DNA/RNA of all genes were programmed by your ancestral urges to exist at all costs. This command directive doesn't ask you to behave. It demands you to behave. The genes command. They say, "You are directed to protect and defend this unit at all costs and if you do not, you will receive a punishment of pain and be riddled with chronic disease." You have inherited these genes and their directives plus the ancestral traumas acquired and passed to you from your genetic family lines.

It is natural to avoid accidents and hurt because they are against our prime directives of life. When you get into these experiences, you are therefore, in the eyes of the genetic blueprint, wrong!

To be right, you must behave yourself. You must avoid having collisions with the environment that knock you into insensibility. You must not collide with objects that will then impact their energies against your body, mind and spirit so as to confuse your ability to recall them.

So after an accident, a reminder tells the mind and body, "Oh no, he's at it again!" The mind and body think you're going to do it again. They think that you're going to have the same accident again because the event, brought on by the reminders, is being replayed in the mind. And this occurs even if you consciously do not want it to. The mind and body think that you will get into trouble and will try to help you to get out of it. This is the basic fear reaction.

I'm sure you've heard of someone who is said to be "accident-prone." Such a person continually repeats the "bad" behavior. They don't want to have a repeat accident but they are stuck in a sequence, stuck in a trauma.

Why do the body and mind keep reminding the person of the same confused situation? Doesn't it realize the person doesn't want to get into an accident?

No one <u>consciously</u> gets into an accident. Accidents and bad times happen <u>unconsciously</u>. And remember you may be operating under the influence of ancestral traumas as well.

Pleasure is orienting to the individual. Pain is <u>disorienting</u>. In other words, pleasure circumstances add to the awareness of the individual while unpleasurable, painful experiences do much to confuse and beguile him.

What does SAF have to do with this?

The SAF program is constructed to read the status of your memory banks to see how much trouble you may have caused yourself. SAF is like a searchlight in the cave of your mind. It helps you to see yourself better. It finds those places that harbor reminders of events and incidents that have traumatized you.

How does SAF work?

SAF identifies the trauma, tracks where the energy is stuck and finds which organ systems are affected. SAF helps areas of the unaware, unknown parts of your mind to become known again and appreciated. SAF utilizes standard knowledge gathering devices such as blood and urine tests, questionnaires, infrared detection, voice print analysis, biofeedback data and many more to create a chain link of numbers for each particular science.

The numbers that are presented in an SAF chain are readouts of your memory banks and the intensity of the pressure.

An example of an SAF chain of numbers is:

8-3-5-4-11-19-21

In SAF, we assign importance to the numbers so that they can make sense. The significance depends upon the science that is used to describe the number sequence, for example the emotions, fears, organs and glands, etc. As mentioned earlier, SAF takes into account 880 different areas. In the designation of psychology, the numbers of the above chain relate to a time when a person had particular emotions or feelings.

Reading from left to right, the first number (lead) is called NOW and the last number

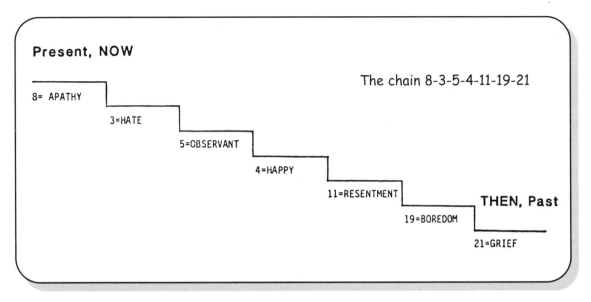

The SAF numerical chain is a layered and stratified history of a person, giving the present time on the left side of the chain and the past on the right side.

on the right (anchor) is labeled THEN. Remember that the numbers are a sequence of importance and a chain link of TIME. By looking at the following time link graph, we can get an idea of the nature of the trauma and when these sequential events occurred.

The lead tells us about the present time, in this case the person is presently apathetic (8) about his situation. Before this he hated someone or something.

The subject of this chain can be found in the middle, or core number. In this case it is about happiness (4).

The anchor is in the past. It is the first step on the chain link of experience. It is the first incident, event or accident that occurred in this sequence and represents the value of pressure that shows how much intensity is on the case. The anchor, grief (21), holds the key to unlocking this chain.

To read this whole chain sequence from the past to the present (right to left) this person first experienced some grief, then boredom, followed by resentment, and so on up the line to the aforementioned present condition of apathy.

The SAF chain can be read like a sentence of this particular person's trauma. It is tailor-made with specific meaning for the person it depicts. The balance of this book explains how to read SAF chains.

Your own SAF chain will only be significant to your particular trouble. Once finding your resistance and traumas, SAF allows you to approach these barriers repetitiously until they are totally dissolved.

How can I find out what my numbers are?

In this book you will find a CD-ROM that contains the SAF Stress – 120 Questionnaire for emotional issues and is an excellent method for finding a chain of numbers. Once you have completed reading this book you will have a better understanding of how to read an SAF chain. This section, chapter 1, can then be used for a quick refresher.

The SAF Stress-120 Questionnaire is a subjective test, which means it works on the basis of input. It will present your viewpoint, your reality as you see it. This particular questionnaire is geared toward the emotional issues each of us faces in our everyday life and the results will be a customized evaluation.

Your answers will be put in order of priority and the SAF chain will reveal hidden, probable causes. It will take what you do know about yourself and help you learn what you don't know about the causes and earlier events that created the situation you find yourself in today.

Those who work with people say SAF helps them get to the main issues in a few minutes, where it previously might have taken a year of work. SAF has been able to unmask symptoms and reveal some astounding information.

By filling out the questionnaire, YOU give the input. And YOU will uncover the answers for yourself. Not only will you discover a new understanding and greater awareness of your traumas and barriers, but also you will get back self-determinism and a sense of self worth. In the process you will free up energy (that has been stuck in time) and will feel revitalized.

Your health and well being have always been your responsibility. Through the self awareness techniques of SAF, it is possible to know yourself. It is possible to find answers.

Once you have the understanding and the knowledge, it is easy to find the remedy and make the correct decision.

> *"The sole purpose of human existence is to kindle a light in the darkness of mere being. Just as the unconscious affects us, so the increase in our consciousness affects the unconscious."*
> — *Carl Jung*

The Goal of the Self Awareness Formulas

The goal of SAF is to move in the direction of Übermensch, to raise the awareness and consciousness level of every man, woman and child. This is accomplished by raising our awareness of symptoms. Most physical diseases have underlying emotional and spiritual causes; some may be very deep indeed. So it is this aspect of the person that we address in SAF. In this way, the immunity level is raised.

With the SAF methods we can:

➤ find psychosomatic causes and trace this back to its source

➤ recognize and eliminate the devastating effects of traumas, dysfunctions and disorders

➤ learn how acquired patterns from a past forgotten trauma can create emotional instability today

➤ discover the startling information on the inner connections of body, mind and spirit

➤ find practical ways to implement this new knowledge into our lives

When we make peace within ourselves, our immunity level rises on three levels – body, mind and spirit. As a result of our own work on ourselves, our family members will benefit, our business life will be more satisfying, and the community of mankind will be more harmonious.

"By using my method of pinpointing psychosomatic causes and tracing this back to the source, we can now understand and eliminate the devastating effects of traumas, dysfunctions and disorder." — Joseph R. Scogna, Jr.

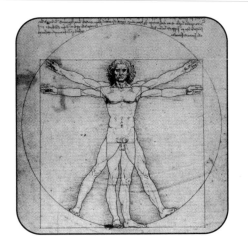

Chapter 2

Anatomy of a Disease and Rapid Aging

In This Chapter

➤ Energy is created by patterns of experience
➤ The mechanism of similars
➤ Body, mind and spirit must be synchronized
➤ Prevention of aging
➤ Origin of Life Energy
➤ The sun's role in Life Energy
➤ Aggressive energies do the most harm
➤ Mental negativity: the most potent poison

Loss of Energy

An individual must make certain that he has enough power to offset the interference of a disease. The energy of all humans comes directly from a blueprint of the genetic matrix; this matrix contains the exact memory traces that induce power or energy. If these circuits become confused or interfered with in any way, the individual's energy is cut to that degree.

In other words, we don't actually "use up" energy. We have an infinite amount of power and energy in our system. We might have the problem of not being able to access our energy banks as when a disease process intercepts the corridors of energy normally used. This is a different view of a disease. Many people have the idea that energy is being drained out of them, when in actuality, there is an agent, an entity or some casual effect interfering with our ability to reach down inside the cell and pull energy out of a vast warehouse of power.

An individual must make sure he has enough power to offset the interference of a disease.

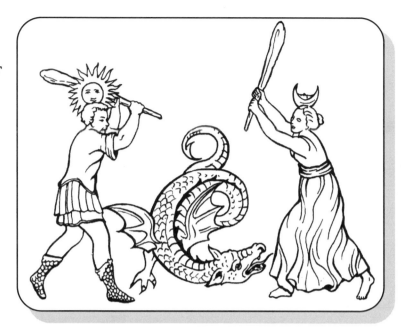

An Individual is loaded with Stored Energy Patterns

Stored energy patterns are facilitated by our ability to experience the digestion or absorption of energy patterns in the environment through food or through activity, enabling us to access those particular energy banks that are native to our genetic structure. It is only when a structure from the outside, such as a food or a toxin, becomes disharmonious with that energy pattern that interference with our energy absorption results.

The actual blueprint of energy can be added to through experience. The genetic structure compiles coded symbols of actions within its memory banks so that we can access these banks and gain energy.

Energy is created by Patterns of Experience

Many people don't understand what energy is and therefore have a difficult time identifying how they "lost" it. Energy, as defined in Webster's dictionary, is "the ability to do work or perform functions." This definition, however, falls short. It doesn't help us understand the composition of energy. We can't get a better understanding of energy by this definition alone. We must look intrinsically at how energy is created. As we study Life Energy and energy related to the spiritual aspects of an individual and the mental capabilities, we learn <u>that true energy is created by the pattern of experiences impressed upon the cells of the body, the mind and the spirit</u>.

For example, if you wanted to learn to fly an airplane, you would have to go through all the motions to learn all the patterns of flying. You must input them into your memory banks so you would have the energy (knowledge) to be a pilot. If you were suddenly thrust into the cockpit of a 747 without having learned these patterns, and were asked to fly that bird, your energy would most likely shut off. You would become terrorized and frozen. You wouldn't be able to move. The energy would be completely drained from your body. If that airplane were to take off with you in it, the only way you could possibly escape death would be to access a memory bank that was similar to the airplane's function and this would permit you to get into action and fly it.

But don't run out and try the plane experiment; there is a simpler, safer test. Ask someone a question to which he doesn't know the answer. Or ask him to define a word he doesn't know. His mind will draw a blank. He will try to fit the pattern of the word into other words he has heard that are similar so he can go into action and come up with an answer. Or show him Greek or Hebrew words that he's never seen. The mind will freeze at the sight of the strange characters, and if he focuses on it long enough he will go unconscious.

This occurs because we can't draw power or knowledge from unfamiliar words. We draw our power from <u>learned memory patterns</u>, and the body draws its own power from learned memory patterns in the genes. The only way to actually stop a person, to make him have the idea that he is "out of energy" (which is an impossibility because energy can't be destroyed), is to mix his memory patterns with strange patterns he doesn't understand.

Energy is created From a Starting Point

It is essential for us to be able to access a location. Energy is always created from a starting point so we must have a stable home base. If we don't have a stable base, we appear to lose energy. The energies in the environment can more easily interfere with our database if we are always on the go. As an example, when you are away from home you have probably noticed that your energy is less coordinated than when you are on a solid home base. This home base doesn't necessarily have to be where your family is located, but it must be a nice, safe place from which to operate. It must be an area where you can allow

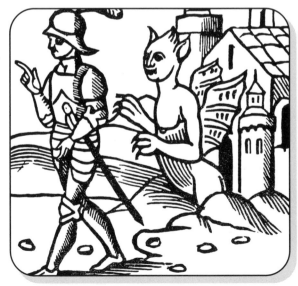

Energies in the environment can more easily interfere with someone who is always on the go.

your energies and your mental image patterns, which provide you with energy, to roam freely. If you have interference, such as the kind of opposition found in a crowded house or with familial tensions, you will lose power. In this case, it is very easy for you to gain back your energy. You merely need to withdraw from the offending energies that are moving into your system and interfering with your mechanism. This withdrawal allows you to reach into that endless pod of energy inside your mind and your genes. Many people can be saved tremendous hardships by just moving out of the environment that creates this incredible phenomenon of energy starvation.

Energy Must Be Free Flowing

If energy is utilized improperly or out of sequence, it will break down. Even if a person can access his memory patterns of energy, if he uses these incorrectly, he may double back on his own power to make it interfere with itself, just the way a garden hose can be knotted and thus impede the flow of water.

An Endless And Timeless Power Pack

The greatest power that is given to an individual is his ability to absorb energy from his own system, an endless and timeless power pack. If he doesn't know the exact formulas for extracting energy from his memory banks, he will wind up with the primary phenomenon of disease, which is loss of energy and loss of the ability to think. His energy will move into a state of confusion. He must learn the formulas for sequentially extracting energy from his system or he will remain obstructed, impeded and suppressed.

The Mechanism of Similars

One of the most important actions to understand is the ability of the human system to translate one pattern for another. This is the mechanism of similars. A person can move very handily in a new situation if he can compare the new situation with similar ones in his memory banks.

To return to the airplane example, there was a well-publicized incidence of such a transition. A passenger had his first flight lesson in the air after the pilot suffered a fatal heart attack. As the passenger sat in the cockpit looking at the lights, dials and strange controls, nothing looked familiar. A second pilot flew his plane behind the distressed airplane and was able to talk the passenger successfully through the landing process. He did this by getting the passenger to look at the panel of the airplane as if it were a car dashboard, to see that the yoke was similar to a steering wheel and the controls had similarities as well. If the passenger/pilot had not been able to make that transition of similars, then his energy would have been frozen, blanked out and missing. All the people in the plane would have died. But because this passenger had the ability to translate energy into similar patterns, he was able to act appropriately in this terrifying situation.

Disease Entities Use Similars

The use of similar patterns can also be accomplished by disease entities when entering an individual's system. In fact any similar energy pattern can move into a person's body and disrupt his energy by confusing and beguiling his system.

One good example is the chelation of minerals. The human body has the capability of knowing every substance that belongs to it and this makes it very difficult for a person to absorb certain minerals. Manufacturers, in an effort to gain greater absorptive power for their products, disguise the metals in a chelated form. The metals are enclosed in a structure of protein so the body believes it is a protein and thus accepts it. By this method of creating a similar, the body is tricked into absorbing the metals.

Similarly, a disease entity can chelate itself and fool the individual's protective mechanisms into letting it inside the body's sacred guarded areas. Many of the powerful diseases such as AIDS, polio, and other contagious illnesses have this same mechanism; they trick the body into letting them inside by disguising themselves as friends.

Body, Mind and Spirit must be Synchronized

A person can easily destroy his body with his mind. A greater percentage of illnesses are psychosomatically caused rather than created by physical means. It probably occurs in the same ratio as airplane crashes; pilot error is almost 99% the cause of crashes while the actual physical structure of the airplane is much less often to blame.

The human body's pilot – the mind and spirit – is almost 99% to blame for mishaps. The body itself is such a miraculous mechanism that it could extricate itself from almost any kind of danger or trouble. So, it is very important for those who seek increased energy (health and well being) to make certain that body, mind and spirit are synchronized.

Unsynchronized Body, Mind and Spirit Energy Creates Disease

If the energy patterns are not matching, there will be trouble. For example, if you are performing grueling mental work and you forget to eat, you will wind up "eating your body," or chewing through your energy stores. The mind, when learning and accepting a lot of information, is also programming these bits of data into the genetic structure. This action causes a depletion of energy because the mind's mechanisms are interfering with the old, known patterns of the body. The body must catch up, so to speak, and assimilate this information so that it can implement these actions. For instance, you can very easily learn the rules of basketball from a book, but when you first play the game you'll be very clumsy and sloppy. This is because the body has not been programmed with the messages the mind has learned from the book. It takes time. The body must be inscribed with hard work, practice and exercise.

The entire phenomenon of this connection between the mind, the spirit and the body is the basis for all upsets and diseases. When we are out of harmony with our own system (either body, mind or spirit) we create more trouble for ourselves than any kind of offending substances in the environment ever could. The familiar saying "man is his own worst enemy" is very true. Once we learn how to harmonize our training with body, mind and spirit, we are much more adept at being able to control invading forces from the outside.

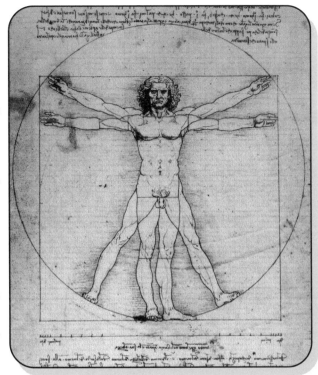

Vitruvian Man, 1492. This illustration has come to symbolize complete health of body, mind and spirit. But in fact it is a depiction of the principles of Vitruvius, Greek philosopher of the 1st century BC. Vitruvius wrote that his ideal, well-rounded man would have knowledge of writing and drafting, natural philosophy, medicine, law, astronomy and mathematics. These principles were revived during the Renaissance and have been immortalized in this illustration by Leonardo da Vinci.

Prevention of Aging

The human being's system must be protected at all costs. It must build a barrier against invading ideas that are not consciously understood by the body, mind and spirit. In effect, if we wanted to exist forever, we must never let anything come in that is unknown. We must never let blackness enter our field of light, for this is unconscious information moving into the known system. It may interfere with our most precious energy sources, the wells of power that have been built up from generations of existence.

Origin of Life Energy

"From where does energy come? From where does a human being take his Life Energy?" These questions have been asked frequently at lectures and seminars. Few people realize that energy is passed on from cell to cell, from one generation to the next; energy is part of a tremendous process that originated with the first inscription on planet Earth. Humanity and all life have experienced this cellular engraving over and over again. It is a present our parents gave us at birth, but we must take care of this present and nurture it.

Genetic Code Must Be Learned For Infinite Power and Energy

If we don't learn the genetic mechanisms that have been bequeathed to us, they will <u>consume</u> rather than <u>give</u> us energy. As a result, the process of aging is programmed into mankind.

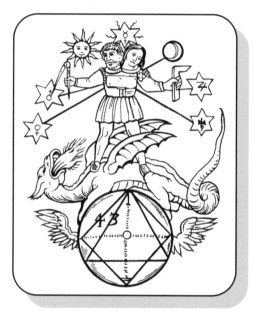

Once we learn the genetic code inscriptions, we will have an infinite source of energy.

It is the ultimate goal of a person who is using sophisticated symptom and self-awareness programs (SAF) to understand the basic inscription of the genetic codes. Once we learn these inscriptions, we have an infinite source of energy.

Life is a blueprint and a mechanism; a genetic challenge that enables each of us to carry out our particular codes or program. If we don't heed our program, we will die from it, for it seems the genetic codes have allocated only a certain amount of time here on Earth, and only so many memories are allowed to escape the energy pod upon which we draw energy.

The Sun's Role in Life Energy

This genetic mechanism takes its cue from the sun, and so we have to obtain an understanding of the exact relationship of the sun to our body. If you believe that the sun is just a pretty orb that shines in the daytime to provide warmth, then you are far behind in your quest to know the human machine.

Earth's Resistance and Ohm's Law

Planet Earth has been endowed with the sun's light. More than likely, the Earth started as just a point in space. This particular solitary energy point resisted the sun. As the sun irradiated the Earth there came a great energy struggle. This energy struggle produced the fire that molded the planet into position.

The most basic electric laws on the planet Earth provide an understanding of this resistance. It is called Ohm's Law. It states that every energy in the environment will meet with an opposition or a resistance. This basic law, which must be obeyed, is programmed into every human being as well.

The Sun Clock and Genetic Timetable

The genetic structure, over eons, has programmed a human being to pay attention to the cycles of time. We are given only so many days and these days number close to 25,000 for a full lifetime. Each one of these days has a specific amount of radiation attached to it. It is one day of the sun – a sun-day – and as the planet rotates, the sun sprays its energy upon the inhabitants and each one of them is nourished by it. Each one of them receives one more push or step forward on his genetic program. The genes respond in kind, for they are, according to Ohm's Law, called a resistance. Each time the sun crosses the sky, another arbitrary "click" is triggered in the genetic structure, and another digit is added to the genetic timetable, which is the aging clock for a human being. As people age, they never realize that if they were to let go of the resistance, to eliminate or vanquish the resistance, they would stop aging. Theoretically, they would never get old, they would be whatever they wanted to be; they wouldn't have to follow the preprogrammed timetable that has been provided for them.

However, the sun is a very formidable power. Its intense heat and tremendous energy create a subtle apathy. In one sense, a man is certain he will be here every day. In another sense, he acknowledges his eventual fate in the same way he observes the growth and decay of vegetation. A kernel of corn grows into a beautiful stalk and produces a ripe fruit, but as it is exposed to the sun over and over again, its own genetic

Life Cycle

37

program causes a treacherous-looking demise. The living corn wilts, decays and loses its precious fluids.

It is observable that the human being will follow the same actions. We will grow strong and reach maturity only to wither and die. Mankind has reluctantly accepted this as fact. It has been programmed into our cells. In the course of a lifetime, human beings struggle against the program. We fight and kick by using drugs, poisons, herbs and all manner of psychic and physical remedies to get away from this blueprint.

Deities, Saints, and Saviors: Breakers of the Genetic Code

No one has ever beaten the prime genetic blueprint except those considered deities, saints and saviors. Homage is paid to these individuals because somehow they have broken the genetic code; they have seen through it. The funny thing is, there is never a penalty for understanding the genetic law. As a matter of fact there is a reward: eternal life. By understanding the genetic code, a person escapes dying in a feeble state of unconsciousness; he escapes from never really understanding from whence he came.

SAF – The Key To Unlocking Genesis

Today the SAF program of self knowledge awards this genetic information, this ability for understanding the connections of body, mind and spirit, to the population. Just as Prometheus took fire from heaven and gave it to mankind, the SAF program is bequeathing these genetic secrets to the human populace. Because poisons are completely corroding this planet, and background radiation in the environment has increased ten fold in the last 40 years, it is imperative to use a tracking system that will detect radiant sources that push the organs and the human body into a more rapid status of decay. It is the author's wish that individuals learn more about their own systems. When it is their time to die, they can do so peacefully and more consciously. It is the author's desire to impart this information so that an individual doesn't have to leave this earth plane in mis-

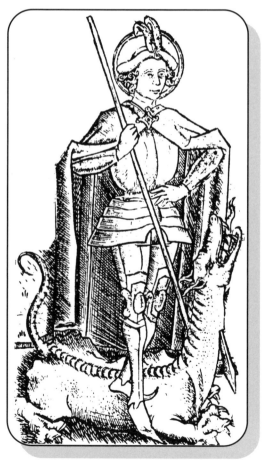

St. George slays the dragon.

ery, misery that comes primarily from misunderstanding.

All That Exists Was Once Sunlight

What causes aging and dying? Is it really just the sun? If this is so, then how can some people sit in the sun all day and be nourished?

The sun has a particular function in relation to the hormonal balance of the individual, and the irradiation of sunlight on the skin produces the much-needed vitamin D for healthy bones, teeth, and energy. It is actually the planet's hidden energy sources, which were once of the sun, that interfere with the human being.

We must recognize that everything that exists on this planet was once of the sun. Trees, animals, even the rocks were all, over time, fashioned out of sunlight. The relative density of each of these materials, animals or vegetables depends on the concentration of sunlight. The whole scale of life and living things on this planet is essentially a variation of congealed sunlight. Any product that uses energy, especially electricity, is one that has broken up sunlight into its finer electronic parts.

Electricity: Sparks of the Sun

In ancient times, researchers discovered some amazing natural properties in minerals. Thales and Pliny both wrote that when amber was rubbed, this fossilized vegetation had a power to pull things to it. The physician of Queen Elizabeth I was the first to coin the word electric, after the Greek word *elektron* (amber).

Even earlier, Stone Age man had discovered that when he struck a flint rock, sparks were produced. The astute observers at the time noted that when this congealed energy of the sun (quartz) was broken apart, a tiny piece of the sun (a spark) split off from the rock.

In the same sense, the electrical energies that pervade our environment today (appliances, television, radio, microwave, etc.) use tiny split-off sparks of the sun. When a person is near electrical devices these unseen energies can sneak into the body and interfere with the genetic blueprint, disrupting its power sources. Not knowing it, we can become contaminated with this radiation.

It is not enough just to say background radiation increases the daily tally of sunlight; it is the <u>kind</u> of electrical phenomenon and radiation (ionizing or non-ionizing) that can adversely affect the human being. These particular toxins and environmental contamination produce all manner of descriptive diseases and leave their own signature on an individual.

Aggressive Energies Do the Most Harm

Basically, it is the aggressive energies in the environment that we would never suspect that do the most harm, causing us to lose our ability to maintain energy and power.

It is very easy to create a scenario of hypoglycemia (low blood sugar), a condition manifested by tiredness, exhaustion and anxiety, by just giving someone a certain amount of X-rays. A much easier test would be to lie out in the sun for six hours straight and receive a severe sunburn. Along with the burn, the feelings that accompany this are exhaustion and weakness, or hypoglycemia. What happened in the second case is the poison of the sun, the excess radiation, has overridden the person's own energy mechanisms. From both X-rays and the sun, the person will remain in the low energy state, hypoglycemia, until he recuperates and gets his energy back.

Study and Track the Offenders

It is <u>vital</u> for us to study and learn all the possible contamination and radiation sources that exist. And then detoxify. If we allow these toxins to sit in our system (often it is unbeknownst to us that we even have any toxins), then we are liable to encounter an energy starvation situation. In addition to the lack of vitality, by not detoxifying you may seem to age more rapidly. Your hair may turn gray faster. Lines and wrinkles may appear. Your bones or muscles may ache or become weak. You may be susceptible to infections or simply have a very low energy status.

Poisons Are Inherited

The real sadness of this predicament is that if we keep specific poisons locked inside our system, they are passed on to the next generation. Part of the problem is that people refuse to look at the idea that such a transmittal is possible. The alcoholic, a syphilitic individual, and many disease states are passed on from one generation to the next. Babies are born with the condemnation of being an alcoholic for the rest of their lives. While giving birth, women with active Herpes Simplex II can blind their newborn by allowing the lesion to rub across the baby's eyes when in that very delicate state of balance. More harmful yet is the genetic miasma passed on to the baby.

> "A life without inquiry is not worth living."
> — Socrates

Mental Negativity: The Most Potent Poison

It may be a more acceptable notion that physical diseases are passed on, but it is often the mental processes, which also lodge their poison, that are not acknowledged or accepted as being able to be passed on to another generation. It is very important that we have that perfect harmony between the mental state of energy and the physically created state of energy in order to avert any excessive aging process.

No matter how many physical toxins are removed, a person who harbors bad or ill feelings, such as hatred, shame, regret and resentment, will be doomed to a rapid aging process. Even though we have cleansed our physical body, we will be subject to the same laws of decay, for the energy of the mind is an even more formidable sun-generated energy. It is the energy of sunlight that gives us the ability to create perfect mental energy pictures.

So, if you hold onto a mental image of an unpleasant circumstance from an argument, upset or confusion with a family member, or if you have lost a loved one and can't come to a resolution in this matter, then you will have dosages of mental radiation that will also adversely affect the body. Such diseases are said to be psychosomatic in origin. It is this type of miasma that can be edited with self awareness techniques.

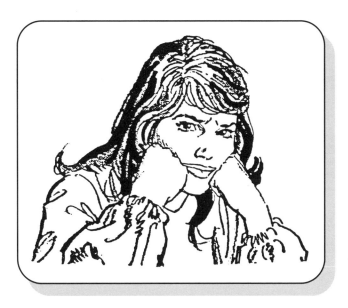

Mental traumas and the resultant negativity will also
adversely affect the body.

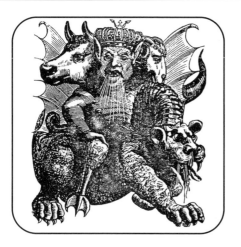

Chapter 3

Discomfort, Pain and Sensation

In This Chapter

➤ How is trauma stored?
➤ How is a past trauma recalled?
➤ Mental attraction and contagion
➤ Immunity on any level – physical, mental and spiritual
➤ How to control the mass, energy and concept
➤ Harmony = energetic power
➤ Confusion = disease
➤ The ability to create

Interference Detectors

A disease situation has its own survival plan. In order to complete its own cycle of birth, growth, maturity, decay and death, the disease has a natural tendency to interfere with the body. Fortunately, the genetic mechanism has already factored in a program to detect when another entity is encroaching on the space of the human body.

Not only does the body have this interference detector, it also has mechanisms to sense when anything is being taken away or stolen from the human body as well. These two detectors are pain and sensation.

Pain and Sensation

It will be noted that when we have continuous pressure on the same area of the system, it will produce pains of various sorts. Those pains are descriptive depending upon the type of entity that produced it. The following is a list of descriptive pains common to humankind: stabbing pains, stinging pains, jabbing pains, searing pains, lancing pains, throbbing pains to name a few.

The difference in the pain phenomena experiences of one individual as opposed to those of another comes directly from the geometric form of the intruder, the entity, and the chemical and physiological relationship of this material to the human being involved. For example, with jabbing pains, there may be some type of energy lodged in the system that is capable of producing a jab; something that has a knife-like quality to it can produce this type of pain. With a pulsating pain, on the other hand, there may be more of an impacted kind of pressure that is rounded on the surfaces. Each person feels pain differently, so in addition to the adjectives, an intensity scale of 1 to 10 is usually elicited to further define the pain that is felt.

The image of a dragon biting its tail was called the Uroborus, Greek for "tail-biter," which symbolized the cycle of death, fertilization and birth. A disease, in its activity to complete its own cycle of birth, growth, decay and death has a tendency to interfere with the body.

While pain is a building up of pressure, sensation is a loss of pressure or resistance. It is space or increasing space. The qualities include dizziness, cold and weakness.

Programs Needed to Detect Pain and Sensation

To understand the mechanisms of pain and sensation, we have to contend with the encroachment of another entity and cope with this particular upset. Any diagnostic program developed for humans in pain or one with power to free us from our disease state must be able to detect when another entity, no matter how subtle, is impinging on any of our circuits. The equipment used to discover the origins of pain must be able to detect this not only on a physical basis, but on a mental and spiritual basis as well.

The program must be able to detect what impinging chemicals, toxins, vermin, poisons or trauma entities may be interfering with the working mechanisms of the human being. It must also be able to uncover losses in the system, such as deficiencies of minerals, vitamins or enzymes in the physical structure, deficiencies of mental capacity, and also deficiencies and losses of a spiritual nature, including those of attitude and consideration. These particular losses could come in the form of personal defeats, such as losing at love and relationships.

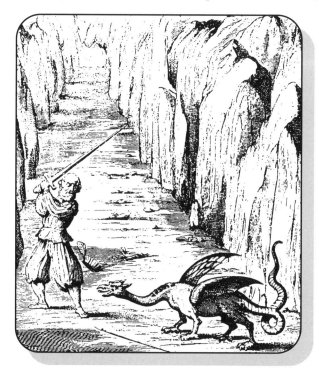

To understand the exact mechanism of pain, one has to contend with the encroachment of another entity on the human being and cope with this particular upset.

The actual detection of the pain and sensations from gains and losses of energy in the system can be easily detected by the buildup or loss of electrical resistance in the system. We experience these losses and increases of pressure and energy by way of symptoms.

It is important to note that each individual disease entity afflicts certain organs, putting heat and pressure on those glandular structures associated with its own genetic and DNA patterns. While pressure is put <u>on</u> specific organs and glands, pressure is <u>taken away</u> from others.

Diabetes, for example, will put pressure on organs such as the thymus, liver, adrenal glands, pancreas and endocrine system. At the same time it is stealing energy away from other organs such as the colon. The diabetic entity is a very powerful one that has been handed down through generations of genetic codes. In other words, human beings have a receptor for this disease. It should be noted that all diseases have their own organ and gland affinities, or organ and gland receptor sites.

SAF has created several different modalities to address symptomatology, including various questionnaires and an infrared detector. The questionnaires rely on the awareness level of the SAFent, while the infrared detector objectively measures the temperatures of venting sites. As heat and pressures build, pain is felt. As cold and loss of pressure is measured, sensations are felt. In many ways the questionnaires are the preferred method. Without an understanding of the SAF numbering system, and with little or no verbal exchange as the infrared operator scans the face, hands, feet or other area, the infrared seems to work "like magic." In this case the operator is the one in control, not the SAFent. This defeats the purpose of <u>self</u> awareness. A thorough understanding of the SAF numbering system is the only thing that is essential for you to increase your self knowledge.

Discomfort, Disease and Dragons

Discomfort felt from a disease condition is merely the entity, or the dragon as it is affectionately called in SAF, encroaching on the human space and taking up root there like a parasite. When this happens, you may think you feel a loss of energy, but in fact it is the aggression, the attack of the entity that is interfering with your ability to reach your own energy pods.

> *Discomfort from a disease condition is merely the entity encroaching on the human space and putting down roots.*

Structure of a Disease

The structure of a disease entity is very simplistic in nature. It is based on a binary system of pressure and space. Its pressures have specific affinities for specific organs and glands, and its spaces are those organ areas that it doesn't attack.

The Dragon Entity Can Change Form Rapidly and Easily

Because the entity changes form, it is impossible for drugs of any nature to cure a disease. There is no such thing as a curative drug for diabetes. There actually are not any curative drugs for any condition. The only "cures" that have any workability have been vaccinations, but even they have fallen short of the mark. This is because the disease mechanism has the innate ability to change itself and alter its ability to produce pain and sensation within the body. This is the characteristic that must be traced and followed if humankind is ever to completely rid itself of disease.

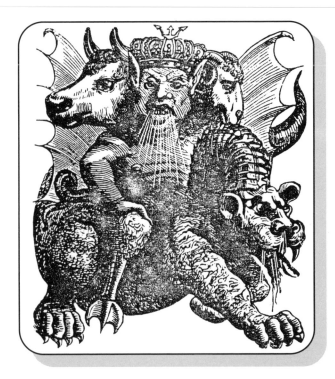

Disease mechanisms can alter themselves and produce pain and sensation within the body.

Disease entities primarily use the nervous system to inflict pain and sensation on the human body. It is the electric character of disease organisms that gives it the ability to change and to aggress against the human state. This is why it is so incredibly difficult to eliminate a disease from the body. When a disease entity is attacked, it can simply change form and turn into another disease.

For example, a person can have a kidney problem or urinary tract infection and very easily, after treating this condition, have it migrate into his feet and cause what we call gout. There are many examples of this kind of phenomenon. Very few people are aware of this mutation process until they've developed cancer and the metastasis is evident; the areas that have become metastasized begin to fester and oxidize.

Disease Entities Are Mental in Nature

It must be understood at this stage of the game that disease entities are wholly mental in nature. Their electric potential is attitudinal only. Diseases themselves have no substance. The actual entity or vortex of a sickness or a trauma is absolutely invisible. In order to activate, diseases must already be buried in the human mind. The disease entity has no wish or will to do harm to the human body, it merely wishes to survive on its own. It sees the body as a feeding ground. It sees an area where it must take up root to survive. It is not stealing energy from the individual, it is just interfering with the human's energy pods.

46

Diseases Have Their Own Genetic History

Disease entities gain most of their energy and power against humankind the same way that a human being acquires all of his energy. Disease entities have their own genetic history. The longer and older the disease, the more formidable it is against humans. Newer diseases are vanquished quite easily, while older ones take up root and with their own genetic mechanisms, foment plans and programs that alter their structures and confuse individuals and scientists into thinking they are other diseases. For example, syphilis may have been stopped by the action of penicillin; however, it may have easily transmuted into another condition called AIDS.

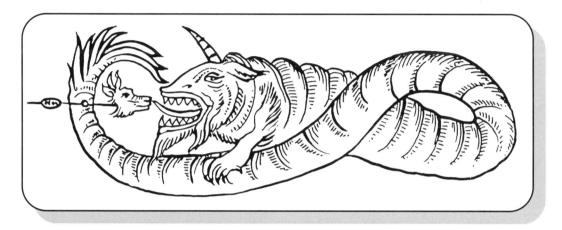

The longer and older a disease entity, the more formidable it will be to face and decipher.

Mental Origin, Stored Trauma

The disease entity itself can't muster enough energy to create itself in a single lifetime. This may be the most fantastic statement that has ever been made about a disease. It must have a predisposed receptor site for which certain environmental toxins have an affinity.

> *All diseases of present day origin have already been logged and catalogued by the genetic structures in the ancestry of the individual.*

It may be the medical breakthrough of the millennia to realize that: All diseases of present day origin have already been logged and catalogued by the genetic structures in the ancestry of the individual. It is a medical fact that a disease process can't initiate without a person having the predisposition or the receptor sites within the body to generate such a process.

There is No Such Thing as A New Disease

Diseases are merely formations or re-formations of the same old characteristic illnesses. The main problem is that we have weaknesses of certain organ structures. These weak organ structures give rise to the characteristic formation of disease patterns. For example, a diabetic will have degradations of the thymus, the liver, the adrenal glands, the endocrine structure and the pancreas. There may also be upsets in the posterior pituitary that control the fluid balance of the body, but this varies depending upon the type of diabetes.

How does Weakness in the Organs begin?

The answer to organ weakness can be found in traumatic experiences that were created in the environment long ago. The genetic mechanisms record everything: every trauma, every brush with danger in the environment, and every upset that may have some bearing on our general ability to survive. This is a necessary survival mechanism so that future generations can concoct systems and programs to avoid these same dangers.

The organs that are the weakest are frail because they have not been able to solve the riddles of concussion that occurred in the past. If we are born with weak kidneys, for example, then some trauma or some upset that happened to an ancestor remains unsolved. It then becomes the task for each of us who are awake and aware in our present day environment to solve the hand-me-down riddle of our genetic structure.

Weaknesses Are Caused By Past Confusions

It is the primary bewilderment of our present day organism that causes us weakness in any zone of our body, mind or spirit. In a sense, when you are born, you contract to spend this lifetime trying to figure out the miasma of your ancestors. This is no errant rule or principle and this is not a process that is mystical; it is an obvious day-to-day, clinically observed situation. A person who acquires Herpes Simplex II at birth will almost certainly deposit or relinquish his segment of this disease to his offspring. Fathers who are diabetic certainly increase the risk of diabetes in their children. Mothers who are alcoholic will have babies who are alcoholic and these babies will have to contend with the added problem of fetal alcohol syndrome.

How Is the Disease Stored as A Trauma?

From the most basic laws of electricity and the phenomenon of magnetism, we can begin to get an understanding of this genetic blueprint. <u>Energy in collision with other energies makes tracings the same way that light from any energy source in the environment can make a photographic print.</u> Mankind has been able to duplicate this process into a startling effect – a photograph. This tracing is the same mechanism used within the human body.

Metals in our system (especially silver, cadmium, zinc and heavy metals) have the propensity to be etched upon the memory banks in particular formations, enough to store the entire content of many of our dramatic life situations.

Does SAF always focus on pain?

The SAF system is able to trace <u>all</u> events. Pleasurable events are stored in one memory bank and the unpleasant events are stored in another memory bank. But all of these particular mental-origin recordings are there primarily for reference and energy.

Remember that we draw all our energy from the genetic mental image banks. It is these energy patterns that give us our power to perform any action. Of course, at the same time, there are dramatic, traumatic mental images etched in the genetic structure that can alert us to danger in the environment or stop us altogether.

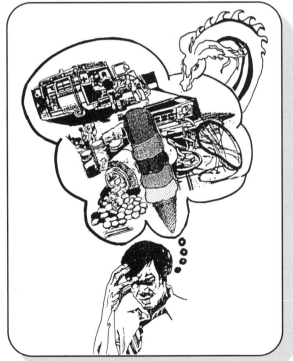

How Is A Past Trauma Recalled?

These mental image pictures are stored in particular sequences, and they have their own ability to be called or recalled for examination. What give them the ability to be recalled are familiar circumstances in the environment. Any particular pattern, sound or color that is present in the environment in the present time has the ability to call up or pull forward for examination images from past genetic stored mechanisms. This is how you obtain power. If your recall system is cued in to pleasant events,

The mention of "ice cream" stimulated an earlier "unhappy car accident." You may be able to see the ice cream cone but <u>feel</u> all the rest of the jumbled sequence.

> *The use of the SAF program is indicated in situations where a person has negative emotional ties that are draining energy in the present.*

then your power will be great. If your recall system is cued in to negative, dramatic emotions and events, then your power will be diminished.

Remember the ice cream cone incident in chapter 1? That would have been recorded by the genetic mechanism as a pleasant, happy event. But after getting the ice cream cone there was a car accident, which would have been recorded as unpleasant, pain, confusion, etc. The pleasant and unpleasant emotions of those events became ensnarled so that the mention of "ice cream" brought to mind the cone <u>and</u> all the darkness of the unpleasant accident. This happens to us on a daily basis, often just below our conscious level.

Present Environment and Past Situation: The SAF Method Finds the Link

By selectively editing such situations, you can gain great power and energy. Otherwise, if you are cued in to an unhappy circumstance in your genetic memory banks (and don't know how to edit these), you will certainly lack the power or the energy to deal with situations in the present environment. If you are able to separate pleasant situations from negative ones, you will be able to operate more efficiently. The SAF method is not a shotgun system; it is a program used primarily to seek and hunt down negative emotional and physical characteristics that haunt you.

The SAF method has the qualities of a screening mechanism. It can filter out the negative situations while leaving the positive ones alone. Some people doing the SAF formats will note that SAF is focusing primarily on negative emotional states; this is precisely why the system was created. Others ask the question "Doesn't the SAF say anything positive?" The answer is yes, it does, in the sense that it will indicate when a negative is lessening. But it doesn't focus on positive circumstances because these don't necessarily need to be corrected. The SAF program is indicated in situations where a person has negative emotional ties that are draining his or her energy in the present environment.

Mental Attraction and Contagion

Throughout the past history of mankind, disease entities have continually infected the human race. However, there is a specific law in the universe that states <u>no two entities can occupy the same space at the same time.</u>

In other words, you will lose power if an entity moves into your space and tries to take up your location. Your power diminishes because the entity is interfering with your most basic energy function: to reach back into the genetic tracing banks and obtain power.

When an infection or virus such as AIDS is able to infiltrate its way into the actual DNA mechanism itself and reprogram it, then the individual will certainly suffer. His body will begin to deteriorate rapidly because he has all but lost his defense mechanism. However, we shouldn't put attention on the disease AIDS as a process that needs to be eliminated. The defenses of an individual with this disease were weakened long before he contracted the disease. That particular genetic line was interfered with over a period of eons, so the virus was able to invade. That particular riddle of defense had not been solved.

It is curious to note that some individuals who have close contact with others who have AIDS have developed a specific antibody; only time will tell whether these people themselves will develop the full-blown condition.

This antibody-type process is effective in vaccination: a certain substance is put within the body to tell the DNA/RNA genetic planning mechanisms the exact blueprinting structure of the offending organism. If we want to gain immunity from a certain disease, we must have those blueprints. If our defense system doesn't have the blueprints, any organism in the environment may be able to attack us.

Immunity Can Exist On Any Level: Physical, Mental or Spiritual

Immunity, in the perspective of SAF, can exist on any level; it doesn't have to be from viruses, bacteria, parasites or physical invaders. There can be immunity from emotional disturbances, addictions, thinking problems, confusion or spiritual distress. The wholistic system – body, mind and spirit – has protective mechanisms capable of thwarting or

> *An entity need not have wings and a long, pointed tale. It is any mechanism with mobility and a pressured environment.*

warding off potential invasions by any entity.

Contagion comes about because 99% of these disease energies are invisible. It is almost impossible to know whether the person next to you in the elevator or across the room harbors some type of gigantic, demonic entity, even if it is able to encompass an area of four city blocks! Those who are aware can sometimes <u>sense</u> such an unbalanced person as soon as he or she enters the room. The poisons injected into the environment by those who harbor such incredible toxins make the world unsafe.

SAF Method puts Light in the Darkness

An entity, in our particular sense, is a complex of energies that is able to cause a situation in the body. It is unfortunate that many people believe "an entity" must have wings and a long, pointed tale. This is not necessarily so. Entities, in the SAF way of thinking, are any mechanism that has mobility and a pressured environment. In this sense, an entity could be a refrigerator, car, airplane, dog or most certainly the memory picture of another individual; these will have a more forceful content when they are of a traumatic nature.

Harmony = Energetic Power

It is essential for us to learn to control the mechanisms that create immunity from contagion, because such powers of energy in the environmental are able to send cross-conflicting signals into the body and reduce its power. The way to gain consistent energetic power is to be in constant harmony with the environment, other individuals and our own body as a whole. The only circumstance that can actually disturb this mechanism is our inability to coordinate and balance the functions of reciprocating energies in the environment.

Confusion = Disease

If you are in a situation that presents a new problem that you can't decipher or if there is a riddle or confusion that is overwhelming, you most assuredly will get the corresponding effect of disease. Tracing the common cold yields interesting information. If you question an individual with a "cold" about his prior circumstances, you will find that he has run into some confusion or upset just prior to "catching" the cold. What he has "caught" is the inability to remain immune from a confusion.

A traumatic situation can also foster a disabled immune system on a psychic level as well as on a neurological level. In this case, the immune system is not able to transmit a signal to the body to keep it intact and free from harm. If you can't solve the passions of your mind, your body will often succumb to the same upsets. The body will mirror these traumas in a very distinct and different way from the energies of the nervous system and the upsets of the mind.

> *The way to gain consistent energetic power is to be in constant harmony with the environment.*

Control the Mass, the Energy and the Concept of the Situation

For example, if you were to lose your job, you might mentally feel tired. Your nervous system might feel empty and your body may feel a "cold" coming on. But there is always a three-prong approach when considering the control of disease entities – body, mind and spirit.

To control the <u>mass</u> of the situation would mean to get a new job. We can't argue with the fact that when a job is lost it creates a financial hardship. The only way to replace or fix this problem is to get a new job. The point being made here is that mass will cure itself in the obvious physical sense. We can see that if you were employed at one place and lost that job, but then become employed at another place and retained the same amount of pay, there would be no harm done on a financial level.

However, it is the <u>energy</u> of the situation that creates a traumatic field. The energy of the new office and surroundings is now different, and you must make that distinction. It is a different location and a different space. There are many differences that fall under the category of energy, and if we don't recognize these very simplistic differences, we will often succumb to disease, because the body is in the "wrong" location. We must be able to be immune to the changes of energy in the environment.

On the other hand, the <u>concept</u> of the traumatic job-loss circumstance is aroused because you may have liked the people at the old job. At the same time, you may have a distinct hatred for the person who fired you. Many concepts are co-mingled with energy upsets and have very little to do with the mass of the situation. If we were merely android bodies with a pre-programmed set of rules and could be interchanged and plugged into one situation or another, such as the way we would replace a picture tube into a television set, then there would not be any problem. But because of the energy and the concept circuits involved in a human being, many different bizarre circumstances can develop.

Infiltration Causes Loss of Energy

The most important factor in the contagion of diseases or mental states is our loss of energy. In this case you lose the energy field and the integrity of your defense. You defend an area in the first place because the more you can keep this area clean, the more power you can generate.

An infiltration, then, is an enemy of a human being. Once the energy shield is penetrated, parasitic outposts or operations of other entities can worm their way into a person's energy fields and slowly create havoc. You will realize, down the line, that your own demise or death can only be brought about by infiltration.

If we look specifically at the death sequence, we realize that many overpowering forces from the environment breach our defenses over a lifetime, however long that may be. We eventually have trouble with sight, sound and memory recall. The body becomes fragile and weak. There are different unseen energies coming between our energy field in the present time and the original blueprint of energy predicted for us by the genetic mechanisms. In the life cycle, we are somewhere between maturity and death.

In other words, the genetic planning mechanism desires that we work at peak performance at all times. There is no real timetable. The truth is, there are plans and programs for dealing with the intrusion of energies from the environment, and it is acceptable to be intruded upon and to be eaten up.

The final degradation occurs when we die and our remains are put into the ground. At that point, of course, all manner of living creature is able to intersect with the energy field of the body and decimate it.

How to Stop the Aging Process

In order to stop the aging process, three levels need to be addressed and cleansed – body, mind and spirit. Eject all of those impurities that made their way into the physical system and put down roots. Once cleansed on the mass side (meaning the body is

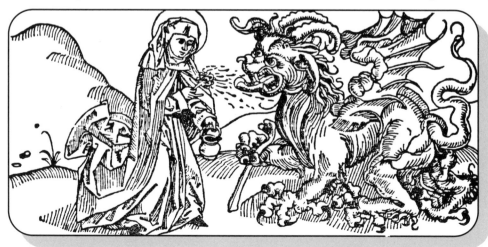

Many overpowering forces from the environment breach the defenses of the individual over his lifetime

completely cleaned out), then the mind should be completely freed of any adverse energy. On the concept level, any erroneous thoughts, concepts, deeds and sins need to be cleansed. In a perfect world, if we were physically cleansed and the spirit and mind were in complete and unreserved working order, humankind most certainly would never die.

The Prospects of Humankind

As this is not a perfect world, we are constantly beset upon by numerous riddles, confusions, foibles and weaknesses. As we grow older, there are so many booby-traps that it is easy to become overwhelmed. Even with the ability and intellect to decipher all or most of the problems of our health, our welfare, and our mental and spiritual state, we find that the ratio of "solved" and "unsolved" is sorely uneven. We try so desperately to figure out and solve a problem or two, all the while we are being overtaken by many more. We may be acquiring one problem per day and only solving one problem per week. With such a timetable and scale, no matter what kind of resiliency we obtain, we will lose the battle. This would be our aging curve.

Of course, in the beginning of life, the amount of confusion is minimal. As these confusions stack up and we gather traumas throughout our life, we begin to observe all the upsets that we can't solve definitively. There are the divorces, deaths, lost loved ones, business losses, things that we are unwilling to tell or share with others, secrets we have to hide, ideas we are unable to communicate, confusing concepts, mental quirks caused by the shifts of energy and location in the environment, and the shame and degradation in our lives.

All those areas where we are unable to recoup our losses will have a traumatic effect. The net result is the inability to discover why. This inability causes us our complaints and grief. It is the intersection of these problems that crisscross the fibers of our being. This intersection of problems stops us from understanding life to such a degree that we are no longer fully alive and aware. We are, more or less, capitulating toward death.

As we become more disoriented and confused in life and less able to be enlightened, we come closer to a death-like situation.

On the other hand, as we become more enlightened and have more understanding, we will live cleaner. The more we let go of what hinders us, the more self knowledge we gain, the more greatly improved will be the quality of our life.

A human being is like a flame. If that flame is able to burn brightly and clear and is filled with understanding, then we will survive well. If darkness covers that light, if the energy is snuffed away from it, if something intersects between the wick and the flame, then the light will be extinguished.

The Ability to Create

The impetus and purpose for all humans is to have the ability to create. We must be able to bring an idea into existence. Day in and day out, we envision what we want in life. If we can't create or envision, we can't produce. If we can't produce, then our ability to see a usefulness for our existence diminishes.

We must see objects appear that coincide with our concept or idea of what should be there. If we want to marry one person and had to marry another, or if we desired one job but settled for another, then we see that our energy was not producing the effects that we had envisioned. This can be very tiring and unsettling.

The disease entity has the same process coordinated with its existence, as does the human being: it needs to create. All diseases that infiltrate the body want to dissemi-nate, procreate and produce. It is not enough for a virus or an entity entering the body to be satisfied with just taking up root in whatever location it finds itself. It must always try to convince the cells and the energies in the body to reproduce its own kind. A disease on a rampage is constantly trying to overwhelm and take over the space of the body.

But even with all the toxins and poisons within our physical structure, we can still be immune to the rampage of a disease. We can add to our immunity on three levels through self awareness and understanding. The greatest and most effective of these are the mental and spiritual levels.

"Man by nature wants to know."
—*Aristotle*

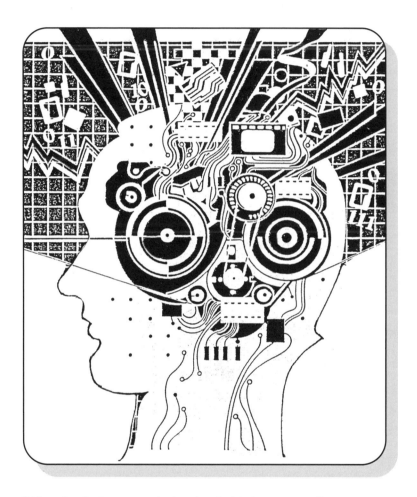

"What lies before us and what lies behind us are small matters compared to what lies within us."   —Ralph Waldo Emerson

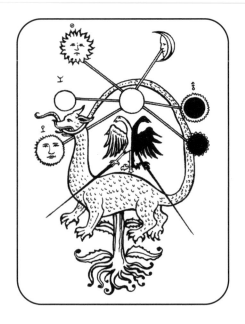

Chapter 4

Numbers, Patterns and Recognition

In This Chapter

> ➤ Mental and spiritual indigestion
> ➤ SAF: a realigning tool
> ➤ Symptoms are signals
> ➤ SAF edits mass, energy and concept
> ➤ Electricity, magnetism, physics
> ➤ SAF numbering system
> ➤ SAF nomenclature
> ➤ SAF and radiation

The disease process is a very specific process of interference by another entity. If a plant has fungus growing on it, we know it is diseased; the fungus is intersecting with the area that should be "plant." In effect, the fungus is trying to take up the same space at the same time as the plant. If we look at a goldfish and see the characteristic goldfish rot, we know there is some entity trying to occupy the same space at the same time as the goldfish.

A similar example would be a human being with dark circles or bags under the eyes, moles, etc. We know he is being intersected by visible energies, and more than likely invisible energies, which are trying to take up the area occupied by this human being.

Creation is a Disease Process

We can observe more parallels in the environment. The actual creation of energy and matter in this universe is itself a disease process. The basic action of survival – eating – explains this concept.

To eat is to ingest, to take in the energies of another. This involution and convolution of substances, which progresses through the entire cycle of existence, is the same process a disease uses to survive.

This may come as a tremendous revelation because people generally think no harm is being done as they eat food. Normally the process is kept under control. However, when the digestive system is not kept under control and you lose your ability to digest properly, you will experience this disease process as if it were a war.

When we eat a food substance, we are attempting to take an existing entity and convert its energies into our own. But if the chicken that is eaten wants to remain a chicken and refuses to become digested or involved in the body processes of a human being, or if the digestive fluids are not correctly in sync to complete that metabolism, then the chicken will remain a chicken. At the same time, it has been cooked, chewed and is inside the space (stomach) of the human. This unfortunate event is commonly called a stomachache, and it is a disease process that can foment problems in the future.

Domestic animals, those that are raised to be food for humans, are more easily digested than wild game. The game often needs to be "tenderized" (beaten with a mallet), or soaked in marinades (enzymes or vinegar) in order to break down the fibers for better digestion. A native, wild trout gives the fisherman more fight than a hatchery-raised trout. The former has a stronger desire to remain a fish, and the difference in the taste of the cooked flesh is obvious.

If we continually have difficulty digesting, then eventually more progressive disease processes will develop.

Digestion: War between Entities

In effect, in the process of digestion, there is a war going on between entities. Each entity is trying to envelop or swallow up the other. The process of existence is a disease, a disease that plagues other entities in the environment as well.

We make it very uncomfortable for the food matter that we ingest because the substances and the life energies that exist around us also want to go on surviving. They certainly don't want to become food; they have their own instincts for total survival. This is one of the reasons why many people have leaned towards vegetarianism.

More highly developed energies, of course, have a greater instinct for survival. Thus, the battle occurs when we must convince another energy that it wants to be assimilated, that it is a lower order of life and would be more suited if it were part of our complex existence. People with weak digestive forces get into metabolic arguments with foods that cause their systems to be constantly in a war-like state.

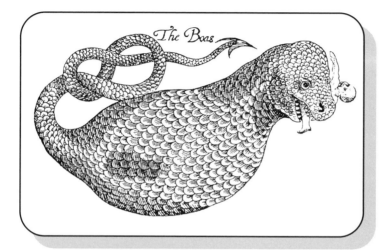

The Boas

The process of digestion is a war in which each entity attempts to swallow up the other.

Mental and Spiritual Indigestion

The same digestive process can manifest itself on a mental and spiritual plane. If we refuse to digest the words, thoughts, dreams, aspirations or desires of another individual, then we may have indigestion of the mind. We could also have indigestion of the spirit wherein thoughts and spiritual ideas enter our space, take up root and infiltrate the whole system. It can happen that we attempt to take on the thoughts and concepts of another, try to swallow them like a tough piece of meat, and are unable to digest them.

Confusion Can Cause Indigestion, Too

For example, you may be exposed to a trauma, death or separation from a loved one, or you may have stumbled onto a situation or event too difficult to grasp. Often these misunderstood situations involve loss, especially when you have attempted to bring about a specific change in the environment or create something and it has been thwarted.

If you envisioned being happily married with children and your partner is unfaithful, this can wind up causing a condition where you have indigestion of the soul, the spirit, and the mind. You can't "digest" or understand how your partner could do this. You will experience the same symptoms as someone with physical indigestion.

It is interesting to note that people who have these confusions and conundrums in their minds as a rule do reflect this to their body. They will have stomachaches, pains and upsets that radiate to the body to express the confusion. For this reason, in America today, there are many individuals with severe digestive problems. Much of it is not from a physical cause but rather a mirror of psychosomatic illness that emanates from indigestible ideas.

Disease Process in the Environment

Again, we must look closely at the environment to see what it teaches us about our own disease process. There would be no such thing as disease if it weren't coming from the master blueprint. In this master blueprint of the universe can be found the intimate process of convolution, involution, and evolution. We must look at the entire process of the sun, its creation and the cycles of Life Energy on the earth to understand that the process of birth, growth, maturity, decay and death itself is a disease process.

In SAF, when we say disease process, we mean that <u>disease is discomfort, lack of rest, or off the resting-place.</u> On the pain/sensation scale we can see the nature of disease. With "0" representing rest, if any energy is exuded in a positive or negative form, it causes a disease condition.

Increasing pressure/decreasing space.

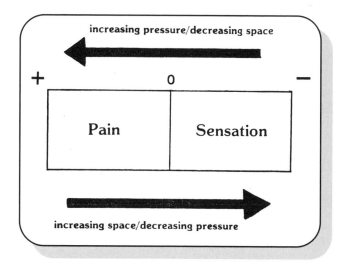

A Disease Represents a Problem to Solve

It is significant to note that the viewpoint of disease is all-important, not just the fact that a disease is created. Diseases are of interest to us because they represent problems that need be solved. It is the reason why humankind exists here on this planet.

If there is any degree of spirituality we must see that our entire existence depends upon our ability to solve problems. We should welcome the idea of having a problem to solve; otherwise, it would get quite boring here on planet Earth and our existence would be meaningless. Anyone who seeks to completely erase, ignore or deny his problems and diseases will have an extremely monotonous life at best.

Countless people have wondered in the past – is the planet Earth a problem-solving location? Or is it created as a problem? The author feels that both are true.

➤ The planet's creation and evolution is the same creation/evolution of the disease process

➤ Disease is the sum total of the processes of learning and understanding

Energies are intersecting one another continually. Even the sun itself must intersect all plant, mineral and animal life on the earth continually to create the cycles of Life Energy on the planet.

SAF: Disease Awareness

So, you may ask, "What does this viewpoint have to do with SAF?" SAF, Self Awareness Formulas, refers to disease awareness. It means to have total awareness of disease processes. However, this doesn't mean that by following SAF religiously you will be completely cured of all illness. As long as we exist on this planet we will have such problems. Disease is the sum total of the processes of learning and understanding. Assimilation of knowledge is similar to the machinery of the digestion of disease conditions and diseased ideas of the mind. Life on planet Earth is a continual process, a journey. Long ago, Aristotle wrote that all human beings, by nature, want to know. There would be nothing to learn or investigate unless a person was diseased, or "off the resting point," in the first place.

Let's look at disease as a process of confusion developed out of an inability to know. The faster we are able to be cognizant, to unravel confusions and mysteries, the faster we are able to eliminate disease. It is that simple.

The slower a person observes and understands diseases, the more prone he is to create long-term chronic conditions. A chronic condition is merely a problem that has gone unsolved for a long period of time. These conditions can become compounded, of course, but this is because we have not been able to solve all of the ancillary riddles of our original problem.

For example, an individual who has genetic "hand-me-down" diabetes has a very difficult problem. He must be able to understand not only his own present day condition, but also the diabetic syndrome that has existed in his ancestors for eons. The same would be true of various cancer syndromes. It is easy to become confused trying to dissect and understand all the ramifications of toxicity that exist in the environment today.

Self Awareness Gives Humanity the Edge

The Self Awareness Formulas were created to give humankind the edge in solving disease processes. As was stated earlier, if you are being invaded at a rate of five disease conditions per day and are able to solve only one or two, then obviously the solution curve is in a downward spiral.

We can observe this by looking at pictures of famous people or movie stars at different time periods in their careers. When we compare the younger images with the older ones, we see that something has happened. When they were young, their bodies seemed to have a smooth and glistening look, and by the end of their lifetimes we can see that there has been a lot of infiltration. Poisons worked their way into each individual's system by different corridors and corners. This is the human condition. In a lifetime, humankind is presented with so many problems, confusions and disease processes that we are unable to solve each one in its proper ratio of body, mind and spirit.

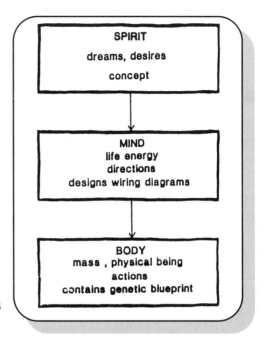

The connections of body, mind and spirit and their control of the genetic blueprint.

There are some aged people who are vibrant, full of energy and it is difficult to tell their chronological age, but many people are so far behind, taking on five or six disease processes or confusions a day that their aging processes become extremely rapid. They are said to be "old before their time."

The SAF program has been developed so we can at least come up to an even par with the number of disease processes that enter our system. When we say, "enter our system" we look at the entire complex system, the mental issues, the spiritual upsets, as well as the physical problems. We can't separate body, mind and spirit. If we attempt to separate this relationship of matter, energy and concept, we will soon realize that it doesn't matter how much mass is handled, how much energy is handled or how much concept is handled. It is the relationship between all three that must be addressed.

SAF: a Realigning Tool

By using the SAF Method, not only will you understand that you have an upset, such as an allergy, you will also understand its origin. This is essential to avoid a repeat performance.

For example, if you have a rash on your hand, you know this rash is coming from somewhere. This rash is mass or matter; it is visible. Remember that visible light is only 1% of the electromagnetic energy spectrum, so when you see a mass, you know that you can edit this mass very easily. You can put calamine lotion on it, soak it or bathe it in Epsom salts.

There are different remedies to use to get rid of a mass; but will it get rid of the total problem? The answer is no, because mass is only one prong of the three-pronged energy system of mass, energy and concept. It will merely bury the problem until it returns in another form.

How Can the Disease Entity appear in a Different Place and a Different Form?

People believe they have taken care of situations (such as diseases) because they have gotten rid of the masses (symptoms), while in fact the energies of the disease roamed freely and turned into other disease conditions. Remember that an entity is composed of energy and energy can't be destroyed.

A person with a rash uses calamine lotion or chemicals to dissolve it. The rash will disappear. But where did it go? Did it go outside or inside the body? More than likely it sank into the body, and the energy that had been routed from the skin and pushed back into the body will now have to find another resting place.

Often, the resting places the disease energies find are more interior, closer to a human organ system. They may wind up in the prostate gland, the pancreas or the liver, and thus add this new extra energy to a vital organ to create a more serious disease problem. Therefore, even simple disease processes, such as rashes, must be handled directly.

Symptoms Are Signals

In SAF, a rash would be considered a signal or a message that some errant energy or mental problem may exist. A person who has a rash can run an SAF program and find out that the rash is coming from an allergy to bananas. A query determines that the individual is eating bananas, so the removal of the bananas from the diet would help greatly. Of course, this again is just shifting masses; it has nothing to do with taking care of energies.

By utilizing the self awareness techniques, we can get to the bottom of why the individual has rashes created by allergies to bananas, and can remove that problem as well. Then the person can eat a banana without getting a rash. This is the basic concept of the SAF Method. It is a sophisticated process that edits not only the mass of the problem, but also the energy and the concept as well.

SAF edits mass, energy and concept

SAF Studies Disease or Discomfort

The study of SAF is the study of life, the creation of life and its disease processes. As was mentioned previously, Life Energy itself is a disease process; it is uncomfortable. If we look at the action of birth, a necessary event for the creation of a new human being, we note a sometimes pain-filled process. This is confusing to a human being. We know that pain is "bad," but at the same time we know that we need it to progress. To repeat a very trite, colloquial phrase – "no pain, no gain."

Throughout all the processes of energy there are sensations and pains. Sensations and pains are relegated to disease processes because disease means dis-ease or discomfort, and that's all it means. We develop disease conditions that we don't understand how to handle, so it becomes a chronic, recurrent condition.

If we understood disease and how it is a necessary function of life, we would be able to put it in its place. However, we wouldn't be eliminating the disease because it exists forever. We would just be changing our viewpoint enough so that we would not experience the problems created by the disease. We would no longer be crushed under by its existence.

Physicists understand that as energy moves out from the sun it immediately creates a disease process on space. As the tempo of energy increases, the rays of energy cause tiny pains (pressures) to the spaces around the sun. This is a universal disease process, but it is a necessary action, one that the universe perceives quite easily and respects in its ability to also create life.

The Sun's Disease Process

The sun's disease process is the simplest disease process to observe. A sunbather who lies out in the sun and overexposes his flesh to this energy for five hours will understand and prove this idea. The burning is proof of the intersection of the energy through space. Once the sun intersects its energy into the human being, the system will begin to blister and decay.

If in the sun too long, a human being's flesh will peel from his body. He has been invaded by the same energy that causes all diseases on planet earth, but it is a disease of which the body is quite aware. On planet Earth, all disease processes start with the sun.

We have learned how to transform the sun's energy processes and develop a viewpoint about it that is non-harmful. Even so, we must have a great respect for this disease process, because the sun has the ability to burn holes in human flesh. If we let this energy intersect often enough, the end result will be skin cancer and cancers of other natures.

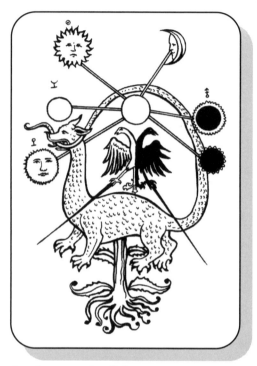

On planet earth, all disease processes start with the sun.

The Age of the Super Disease Format

A simple disease is no more than a simple confusion. Compound those simple confusions and the result is a super disease. We are entering an age of the super disease format – we have less immunity than did our parents and many today are dying of high-tech confusion. Our bodies are becoming intersected, riddled and invaded by poisons that never existed on the planet before. More and more toxins and poisons are being spewed out into the environment, and no one has any idea what kind of effect these will create on a human body now or in the future. The pains, sensations and diseases that come from swallowing, ingesting, breathing or being exposed to such poisons create situations in the human body that are treated by medical doctors with more toxins – the latest sophisticated drugs.

Critical Mass and Spontaneous Combustion

The poisons accumulating in the human system are reaching critical mass. Just like the hydrogen bomb, many people are simply exploding.

The first official incident of spontaneous combustion of human tissue occurred in 1889 when a man driving a milk wagon fell off the wagon and burst into flames. It was a very peculiar incident that no one could explain. Some called it an act of the devil.

In 1933 a second incident was recorded. A woman, dancing in a marathon dance, suddenly caught fire. Observers and crematorium technicians estimated the amount of heat present to be about 7000 degrees centigrade. The dancer was vaporized within three hours.

It was 1953 before another incident made it to the newspapers. This one occurred in Brooklyn, NY. An older woman, sitting in a chair by her window, suddenly caught fire.

When neighbors found her, all that was left were a pile of ashes and pieces of a leg bone. She had been vaporized.

Ever since that incident in 1953, there have been over 750 reported cases of this phenomenon. We can see that spontaneous combustion is becoming more prevalent. It is a high-tech super-disease. There may be different explanations for what is going on in these cases, but it is the author's belief that many of these individuals had been inundated with radiation, toxins and poisons, and their systems reached critical mass.

Accumulation of Toxins Creates Mass

The ingestion of drugs, chemicals, poisons, toxins and hormone imbalances, in association with high radiation sources such as microwaves, X-rays, radio, television waves, nuclear power plant effluence, etc. creates pressure that "goes off" when it reaches critical mass.

This is the same concept needed to create a hydrogen bomb. A hydrogen device contains so much confusing radioactive energy in one place at one time that it explodes. In a similar way a human being becomes angry and "blows his top" or goes berserk and starts shooting people from a tower. This "explosion" phenomenon can be observed in those who have reached their limit, that is, reached their limit of problems and confusions. Again, we have not been able to solve problems fast enough. The problems pile up, we are pressurized and we explode. Spontaneous combustion of human tissue, hydrogen bombs and angry people are similar; what they share in common at the very core is an unsolvable riddle.

Radioactive Elements: Congealed Sunlight on Earth

The sun, constantly baking the earth in its own aura, creates pieces of congealed sunlight on the earth – those coveted elements known as uranium, plutonium and all of the radioactive series. These elements have had so much sunlight, so much energy packed into one element, that they are ready to detonate.

Mankind has succeeded in developing a technology to pack enough of this refined sunlight together until it can't take it any more. It becomes "angry" from the pressure, which causes a chain reaction and it spontaneously combusts.

People have so many disease symptoms, poisons and toxins from being exposed to pollution in the environment, from taking drugs and medicines that they are almost ready to explode themselves. Anything can set them off.

The Primary Grid Work of Disease

The primary grid work for creation laid the foundation for the dissolution of disease.

As was mentioned earlier, the sun causes discomfort; it causes the aging process but it also causes birthing and life. Without sunlight, without the passage of enough sun-days (that is, one 24 hour cycle of exposure to sunlight), a baby would never be born. The baby must complete nine months, approximately 270 sun-days, of gestation. Even though enclosed in a dark womb, it takes 270 of earth's sun-days until a baby's exposure reaches critical mass. In effect, a baby being born explodes out of the womb. It has had enough. It has gotten too big. Its energy has collected and congealed to such an incredible size that it can't exist in that space anymore and it must invade another space. At birth, a baby invades the space of the environment and finds a place outside the mother's body. So, this very important survival mechanism is part of the whole process of causing an individual his primary life discomfort, his growing up. We hear the term "growing pains," but such pains can be perceived as pleasure, depending on our ability to understand the process. It is a matter of viewpoint.

The grid work of the sun (creation and disease) is also the grid work of the SAF method. The power of the SAF method is that it can develop and enhance our viewpoint to explain exactly how a disease process intimidates, and how we can gain back control.

SAF Uses Numbers to Track Disease

The SAF study of the disease process is a universal one founded on the most basic subjects of the universe: mathematics, geometry and physics.

Galileo wrote that the great book of the universe was written in the language of mathematics. Every science must yield to mathematics. The SAF method uses mathematics because numbers are universal to all forms of Life Energy and all forms of disease processes on the earth. Numbers are the triggers for the energy banks. Numbers by themselves have no meaning unless they are assigned meaning. A person seeking answers to complex problems needs to address a wide range of emotional issues, environmental situations and other upsets, and assigning meaning to numbers is the simplest, most orderly way to accomplish this. The SAF numbering system intersects all known sciences and bodies of knowledge, 880 in all. The balance of this text and other books explain fully the numbering system.

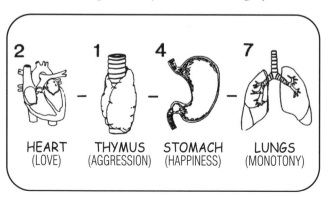

2	1	4	7
HEART (LOVE)	THYMUS (AGGRESSION)	STOMACH (HAPPINESS)	LUNGS (MONOTONY)

SAF utilizes a chain of numbers (2-1-4-7) to represent the organ and gland complex (heart-thymus-stomach-lungs) or the emotions (love-aggression-happiness-monotony).

Electricity, Magnetism, Physics

Madame Curie, Pierre Curie and Wilhelm Konrad Roentgen have contributed to the basic knowledge of the universe. The laws of electricity, magnetism, physics, radiation and gravitation have also found their niche. Max Planck's work on quantum theory ultimately led Niels Bohr, Albert Einstein and Werner Von Braun to understandings that gave us the hydrogen bomb.

Of course, many will argue that because of nuclear madness today, mankind is on the threshold of a nuclear apocalypse. Right now there are tremendous potential hazards with nuclear energy when we consider all the nuclear power plants, submarines, nuclear medicine and the overexposure of radiation in the environment. And a big question remains how to dispose of the partially spent materials whose half-life numbers in thousands of years.

In essence, what scientists have accomplished on planet Earth is the ability to take a piece of sunlight and use it as a thunderbolt. The atomic and hydrogen bombs, as the sun's stepchildren, are not only devastatingly powerful instruments for war and energy producers for peaceful purposes, but have become important study tools to understand more about the human body. Advances in science in the 20th century have given us the ability to understand the energies in and around the human being in far greater terms than was ever before believed possible.

Life Energy Foundation

When I was in my mid-20s, I found myself extremely sensitive to radiation. I had photophobia and a dislike for any type of radiation or heat. TV bothered me. I couldn't go near a radio. Electricity made me jump. The electricity of the car interfered with my energy, and often at night the car lights would go out with a flash. This was dangerous. I was terrified. I had tremendous anxieties and my body felt tired and weighted all the time. I was told I had hypoglycemia and that my life energy was low. In effect, my shields were down, perhaps as a result of the elevated mental/spiritual states of consciousness with which I had been experimenting and then overexposure to radiant energies.

Now, I had been a basketball player and had been in great shape. I was determined to find out what was going on. So my initial radiation studies on cosmic and atomic levels were for my own edification in the hope that I could escape and perhaps control the hypersensitivity. By studying the reports that came out of Hiroshima and Nagasaki, Japan, it was noted and generally understood that the organs and glands degraded in a certain order in the presence of high-intensity, gamma radiation. This sequence, that I later called the Primary Sequence, can be found in *The Threat of the Poison Reign* and *The Promethion*.

In 1979, the Life Energy Foundation was founded. Forty miles away the first nuclear power plant mishap occurred at Three Mile Island, outside Harrisburg, Pennsylvania.

Immediately, radiation was on everyone's mind and at that point I branched out and conducted tests at various nutritional clinics that were springing up all over rural Pennsylvania. All the test data was evaluated under my scrutiny at the foundation. We started a newspaper, *The Life Energy Monitor*, to keep the clinics and interested people abreast of new developments.

Using the Primary Sequence of organ and gland system degradation as the basis of study in the research project, different electronic equipment was utilized and hundreds of composite tests were conducted on human beings with vitamins, minerals, color, glands, enzymes, herbs and other substances. Subjective radiation tests, symptomatology and metabolic health evaluations were composed; out of these were developed the SAF-120 for symptoms, the Stress-120 for the emotions, and others followed (the Stress-120 is included on the CD-ROM with this book). Experimental computer programs were written for analysis of hair, blood, urine, sound, voice and temperature. With all these analyses, it should have been easy to intersect what we knew about the body, mind and spirit connections with what we didn't know and come up with an answer. But something wasn't adding up. After thousands of hours of testing, the computer project seemed at a stand still. It looked like a dead end had been reached. Man's most secret problems, the ones that cause the chronic ills, remained hidden. The continual response seemed to be that body, mind and spirit were vastly too complicated to understand fully and that the actual answers to the confusions of mental trauma connected to body metabolism would remain concealed.

The SAF Numbering System

It took a while to decipher the metabolic codes, those connections between body, mind and spirit. One day, late in the spring of 1980, the first codes were cracked. I had changed the parameters of the study slightly, and my findings indicated there was a Secondary Sequence of organ and gland system degradation. This Secondary Sequence was directly related to radiation acquired from living on planet Earth. This would include the background radiation that is being produced today by microwave towers, nuclear power plants, nuclear testing, radar, metal-smelting factories, auto exhaust, chemicals in pesticides and herbicides, and all the other apparatuses in our modern culture that produce extra radiation. Even the light that is reflected off the moon is included as it has a certain radiational quality.

Another significant code involved the connection of the DNA/RNA and the genetic response to activity and emotion. I had found a way to detect the connection of electricity, radiation and stress to the disease process. Once this was understood, the confusion and fear about sickness and death was dissolved. Those first programs were called *QUIRK – Questions Understood by Intersecting Retrievable Knowledge*.

From that point on, the theory has held up under scrutiny and trials with SAF methods and programming. Diseases and syndromes were continually added to the SAF interface as were the use of different modalities.

"The story of the universe is written in the language of mathematics."
—Galileo

This Secondary Sequence of organ and gland system degradation, and the composition of the particular physical systems is so intrinsically important to the creation and operation of SAF, that without it the method would be nonfunctional.

Understanding the order of organ and gland degradation is essential, for the organs and glands <u>are</u> existence for a human being. They are being affected everyday by exposure to sunlight and radiational energy. Some human organs are stronger than others and can withstand more radiational energy before breaking down. Others fail or age more quickly. For example, the sex organs will fail sooner than the skin. The thymus will fail before the sex organs.

Knowledge of this degradation order gives us the entire secret to understanding the problems, toxins, poisons and all those things that create the disease process. This particular Secondary Sequence and aging process is the formula for life.

SAF Nomenclature

SAF uses its own terminology that best describes ideas and functions that are unique and necessary to its understanding. Those listed here will differ from those found in standard or alternative healing guides.

SAFent: someone who is studying Self Awareness Formulas (SAF) to learn about himself with or without an SAF Monitor. A SAFent is an active participant in the process of self knowledge and enlightenment. The SAFent is not to be confused with a patient. A patient is patient, one who waits, and by definition has already given over his or her power to a practitioner.

SAF Monitor: a person who embraces the principles of the SAF method and techniques in order to help process individuals.

Organs and Glands: Each of the 23 organ and gland complexes in SAF is ranked by number, 1 to 24. Note that the number sequence 17/18 is presented as one number, being male/female endocrine systems with corresponding hormones.

SAF Chain: SAF uses combinations of these assigned numbers, called chains, to decipher a person's case state. Particular sequences have specific meanings. Each study listed with SAF programming (880 in all) has a separate meaning for each of the organs and glands.

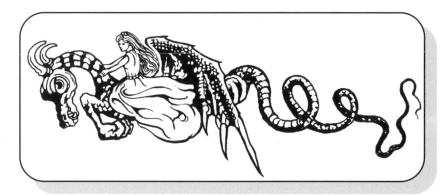

Past remembrances of traumatic experiences that once wrested dragons from their sleep can no longer hurt the enlightened SAFent who can touch and control her dragons.

Emotion: An emotion is a mental experience, which causes biochemical (physical) reactions. We call it an e (lectric) motion. An emotion is assigned to each organ/gland complex. It is often easier for an individual to understand the <u>function of an emotion</u> rather than the function of an organ complex.

Condition: The condition represented by each organ and gland complex aligns its function with the individual's body. The SAF viewpoint gives a slightly different definition than the orthodox view.

Physical and Mental Aspects: Special interpretations are given for the organs and glands in SAF, which help the SAFent better understand the connections of body, mind and spirit.

Reading a Chain: When the SAF Monitor and the SAFent become proficient, the SAF chain of numbers can be read (understood) like a sentence of the SAFent's existence. The chain is a "slice of life" to be examined.

Dichotomy: A division of two opposite but equal sides, both of which give further definition to the universe (the chain) of the SAFent. These opposites enable the SAFent to discern differences, positive/negative, light/dark in the chain. SAF uses 64 dichotomies to add many dimensions to the SAF chain. (The 64 dichotomies are listed in *The Secret of SAF: The Self Awareness Formulas of Joseph R. Scogna, Jr.*)

SAF and Radiation

Again, a distinction is made between the radiation of a nuclear bomb and the radiation that we find on the planet. When evaluating radiation, we must consider all types of energy <u>moving toward the body.</u> Radiation and gravitation are merely fields of energy, and if something is pressing on the body it doesn't necessarily have to be gamma rays, hydrogen bomb particles, or X-rays. In the SAF view, radiational energy can certainly be a pressing problem or a situation that is not understood or is out of control. With the tool of SAF, we have begun to understand how radiational energy affects humankind and how to use that tool to break apart, understand, digest and dissolve a high-tech disease.

But clearly, as the background radiation continues to increase on the planet, this in itself becomes a most compelling reason to study SAF. The SAF method has been created to carry mankind through to the 25th century.

The Axioms of SAF

Axiom 1:

Each of the 24 organ systems (thymus, heart, stomach, colon, etc.) has a life of its own. All are connected to the nervous system.

Axiom 2:

The organ systems sometimes work alone, but many times work in unison with other systems.

Axiom 3:

Various amounts of energy are assigned to the organ systems by the brain/mind complex on a specific timetable.

Axiom 4:

Any extreme stress or trauma such as drugs, operations, accidents, etc., freeze (lock up) a pattern of energy into a non-operational status at the exact instant of impact.

Axiom 5:

Non-operational status of organ systems can be plotted by the special 64 point patented secret mathematical matrix and flow diagram generated by infrared detection.

Axiom 6:

Once detected, the non-operational status can be deprogrammed to a new state of free operation, thereby releasing all injury – past, present and future.

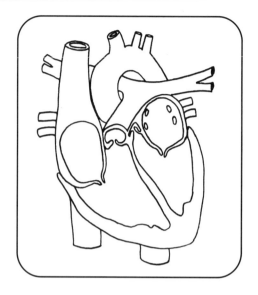

Chapter 5

The Organs and Glands, Emotions and Conditions

In This Chapter

- 1 – Thymus
- 2 – Heart
- 3 – ~~Thymus~~ Colon
- 4 – Stomach
- 5 – Anterior Pituitary
- 6 – Liver
- 7 – Lungs
- 8 – Sex Organs
- 9 – Bones & Muscles
- 10 – Thyroid
- 11 – Veins and Arteries of the Lower Extremities
- 12 – Brain

- 13 – Adrenal Glands
- 14 – Mind
- 15 – Hypothalamus & the Senses
- 16 – Kidneys
- 17/18 – Endocrine System
- 19 – Skin
- 20 – Pancreas & Solar Plexus
- 21 – Posterior Pituitary
- 22 – Parathyroid
- 23 – Spleen
- 24 – Lymph

1

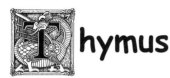hymus

AT A GLANCE:
Emotion: Aggression
Condition: Protection

The thymus gland, situated near the clavicle in front of the uppermost portion of the sternum, is very important to the survival of the body. As a radiation sensor, studies show the thymus gland has the highest sensitivity so it has been assigned the number 1. The word thymus, from the Greek *thymos,* means shield, and by breaking down the word into Latin it is, "shield of the invisible." That is an apt description of its purpose.

The thymus gland is also a monitor for infection and for keeping invaders out of the system. It works with other glands in a network called the reticuloendothelial system, which is cued by the invasion of any entity into the human being's space. The thymus connects itself with the bones, the adrenal glands, the spleen and the thyroid to effect changes in the energy stance of the individual so that he is able to rout out any invading enemies.

If an individual becomes sick for any reason, the thymus gland is primarily at fault. But it is only a sensor that can alert the other organs to go into action. If the sensor is in good shape and the organs that should produce antibodies are not in good shape, then of course, this would not be the fault of the thymus. However, the thymus gland is instructional and tutorial to other glands. It tells the other glands exactly what they have to do to fight off any poison.

When the thymus gland is in very good condition, it is able to read the image of the invading energies in the darkness. Because the body's energy is only 1% visible and 99% invisible, the thymus gland works wholly on invisible radiation.

The thymus gland in the newborn infant is very large, about the size of a plum. As a person ages, the thymus gradually shrinks down to the size of a raisin. Scientists concluded that the thy-

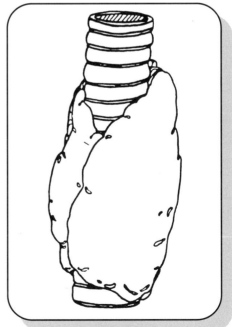

The Thymus

mus gland directed the creation of antibodies, and when it had sufficiently made all the antibodies necessary for a lifetime of defense, it withered away. This was the old and accepted school of thought, but their theory of the withering thymus is an erroneous one. In autopsies performed on athletes, who had been killed in accidents, it was found that they had large thymus glands. The real problem is that the body will collect many more toxins than it can handle so the thymus gets overrun, burning out like fuse. Thus it becomes withered.

The relation of thymus degradation is parallel to the overall history of illness and disease on the planet. Being the first line of defense against infection, the thymus is the weakest in the face of disease. Infection itself has been the cause of the most devastating carnage of humankind in history. In diseases and deaths caused by infection, the thymus is responsible. The Black Plague that spread throughout Europe in the 14th century reduced the population of mankind by 40% within a very short period of time. This was due to faulty thymic action amongst the population and so it has been plugged into the SAF system as the number 1.

Emotion: Aggression

In working with SAFents who had the number 1 appear in their SAF test results, it was noted that not only was there some kind of thymus upset, but also each individual invariably complained of aggression focused toward him or he felt aggressive towards others.

When the number 1 is present, the actions of the person are in a state of overwhelm. He senses the pressure and aggression building up within the system as invading forces intersect with his energy fields. These forces are stopping the flow of energy to organs whose vital functions are necessary for the creation of life. The term aggression is used only with the thymus gland, and is an indicator of thymic malfunction. If the number 1 appears in any SAF chain of numbers, whether found by computer programs or by hand with the questionnaires, the emotion is aggression.

Aggression is the number one trouble of the entire human race. On the national front the most important concern is the protection and safety of each individual and the country as a whole. Man's greatest liability and his greatest foible is safety. So, aggression, used to describe upsets involving the thymus, fits very well into this position.

Condition: Protection

When studying the thymic reaction, we observe the thymus gland's ability to screen out all the unwanted energies in the environment that have a detrimental effect on the human being. If the thymus is run down, it can't come up with the answers that the protective mechanism of the body needs to defend itself. Eventually the body will age and fall apart. As we discover and learn through Self Awareness Formulas, rapid aging is merely a reaction to the intersection of energies that have breached the barricades and the screens of energy around the body.

The whole idea of protection is to thwart or prevent invading forces in the environment from taking over the space that is the body's own space. There are many marauding entities in the environment, and the body has a good index on these. The thymus gland, in association with the nervous system, the brain, the mind and the spiritual aspects, most certainly utilizes this mechanism and its ability to understand an individual's problems in facing a very aggressive environment.

Mental Aspects

In a sense, a person who exhibits aggressive behavior or has difficulty protecting himself maintains a very brittle defensive stance. When confronted he is easily prone to falling apart. Individuals who possess a strong nature frighten this kind of person. When the thymus gland goes out of balance, it is an indicator that there are many unresolved problems on a mental basis as well. Because the mental aspects affect the physical, a person who has not been able to come to grips with his connections in the environment, as far as loved ones and business relations are concerned, will also have stress build up to such a fever pitch that it can automatically destroy him.

Physical Aspects

Fever, pain, swelling and pressure are brought upon the individual when he is infected. It is very important to keep in mind that we can also develop these conditions from a mental stance. A person can break out in a rash from pressure or cerebral upsets. In a physical sense, a person will exhibit definite characteristics. It is an easy task to spot someone with this trouble. The characteristic complaints of pain, swelling, redness, or discomfort in an area is an immediate signal that the individual has a problem involving the thymus gland, that his body is being aggressed against, and that he is losing his safety margin. His protection is in jeopardy. This is obvious in an individual who is nervous and unsure of himself because he is developing a pattern that will ultimately lead him to that critical mass or explosive state. He has to come up with some answers against these toxins and poisons in the environment to stop the onslaught of poisons from overwhelming his body and taking over his space.

2

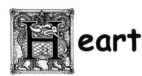eart

In the Secondary Sequence of radiation degradation, the heart is assigned number 2. This organ is one of the most difficult areas in which to control disease in the human being. It is so tangled up with an individual's confused emotional feelings that trouble here can be difficult for practitioners to detect. Radiation toxicity present in the environment has a large bearing on heart trouble. The chest is one of those areas that becomes easily pressurized in the presence of any kind of radiational energy, such as radiation from the sun, from other people, from the environment or from the general pressure and heaviness of everyday, modern society.

The organ itself is a small pump that extends its energies throughout the entire body. According to the Chinese school of thought the heart's actions are the core or operations center of the human being. (In contrast, the Greeks and Romans considered the brain as the center of all existence.)

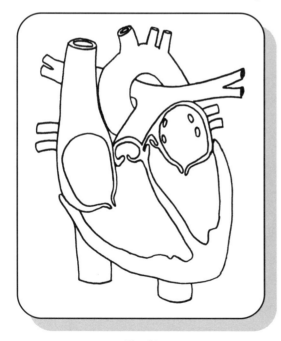

The Heart

The heart has a most resilient crust but it is up against so much stress and degradation during a lifetime that it succumbs to the easy actions of heart-oriented toxins. Heart disease remains the number two killer of mankind, just behind infections and diseases caused by germs and microbes.

Emotion: Love

In the research and development of the SAF program, it was interesting to note that individuals who complained of physical heart traumas (actual heart pains and problems, had bypass surgery, clogged arteries, etc.) also complained of difficulty in their love lives. As a result, the emotion love was assigned to the heart organ. It is not necessary to belabor or prove that this is so, as there are many cases of illness and death due to a "broken heart."

Condition: Synchronize

When the number 2 appears in an SAF chain, it specifically hints at a person's problems with synchronization, meaning that he is not able to coordinate his basic activities properly.

Love has been found to be a mechanism that intersects energies in a harmonic way for greater synchronization. In this sense, love becomes the opposite of disease.

The importance of love is that it establishes a connection between one individual and another; the energy of the combination is greater than either could produce singularly. That is love. If love doesn't happen, it is because an individual is not able to communicate his ideas to his partner or there is some breakdown in the assignment of needs and wants between two parties. Harmonization is necessary. When the number 2 appears in the chain, there is some dis-synchronization in the body, mind or spirit and disharmony in connection with certain people. A disease state exists instead of a love state.

What confuses humankind so thoroughly is the fact that people who attempt to play at the game of love often wind up with a diseased state.

A divorce is a diseased state of love. In this case, love started out trying to cross connect two human beings into a circuit that could have become very powerful and harmonic, but some essential points within their existences were never clarified. It is the darkness of misunderstandings that can overshadow the energy of love.

When the intersection of another's energies into your body, mind and spirit becomes a disease instead of love, it becomes an involution instead of an evolution. If a person stops evolving, if the intersection of your energy with another's stops becoming productive, then you must caution yourself that you are entering a disease zone. Poisons are beginning to build up between you two.

We must not look at love only on the basis of two individual human beings. There could be love between a person and any animated or in-animate object on the planet. This love is the same emotion that calls out for synchronization. It is the love that creates a bond between two entities in the environment that is productive instead of nonproductive. Looking at disease as a nonproductive state and love as a productive state, we can see the dichotomy betwixt the two.

How does this affect the heart? It is curious that those who present the number 2 as the very first number in the SAF chain also had difficulties with disharmony, unsynchronized feelings, low productivity and disease. With the heart in this position (the very core of the individual according to the Chinese philosophers), it begins to decline. It is time for an individual to spend his energy searching for a common denominator in the environment that will help him become more productive. It is time for him to patch up communications between himself and his loved ones. It is time to find the proper people to create a union that will lead to a harmonic state. Only then can productivity survive.

Mental Aspects

It is extremely important for the mind of an individual to remain organized. When confusion sets in, disease runs rampant. The synchronization and attunement of energies in the mind and spirit are necessary to coordinate the true inner feelings of love that affect the heart. If you have no ability to communicate your feelings to your partner, then the relationship must surely suffer. It is herein dictated that if you want to cure your heart you must first cure your mind by dissecting your confusions on the most basic levels. You must begin to educate yourself on how to communicate and how to accept the realities of another so that you can have great feelings of love and appreciation, if this is a goal.

On the other hand, if you hope to squash any connections between human feelings and believe that you can exist on your own, then you don't need these messages. You must effectively shut yourself off and need not communicate. You must not show anyone you are able and willing to create bonds necessary for greater productivity.

But if you are genuinely interested in becoming more able and more powerful, you must intersect your energies without creating disease. The only way you can do this is with the love process, which is born of synchronization. The give and take of life and energy must be there.

Physical Aspects

People are not always able to understand the feelings that come between two people. Are the feelings disharmonious or harmonious? How can I detect if my relationship is actually creating a disease process? If there is a connection between two people, and productivity between these two people is diminishing, or going into nonexistence, then you must re-evaluate or re-examine what this connection is with that other individual. It can't be love. It can only be a feeling that is confused with love.

It is essential for any student of SAF who desires to learn these powerful research findings to know that throughout the development of SAF, each person has voiced the most incredible and profound thoughts and relationship to his disease state. These statements by individuals (their complaints, worries, troubles, etc.) are vitally important; they will allow the rest of mankind to escape the miasma of chronic disease. We must be ready and willing to confront all that the environment has to offer. We can't deny or disavow any action of which the human body is capable.

The reader may wonder if the author has strayed from his scientific studies in this discussion on love. This is not so. The important thing to realize about energy is that it takes on many different forms. If we are not able to recognize and accept what we can create, then we surely are missing something. It is the idea of SAF to allow nothing to go undetected. Therefore, it is important to confront and observe all the phenomena associated with energy, and all the possible conditions that can exist. Once we are able to do this, a disease will not be able to escape our understanding.

3

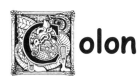

olon

AT A GLANCE:
Emotion: Hate
Condition: Detoxify

The colon, or large intestine, is situated in the lower half of the body in the abdomen. It is the final segment of the alimentary canal, extending from the cecum to the rectum. It absorbs water, minerals and other materials, salvages these from the digestive process and then discards the unwanted matter. When the colon is in good working order, it creates some necessary nutrients, filters poisons out of the body, and in some extreme cases saves an individual's life.

What the human being doesn't realize is that he puts substances into his body that act as spies and double agents. Anything eaten that can't be absorbed or digested becomes a toxin. It becomes a toxin because it now has intersected its energies with the body's and has been allowed to come into the system beyond the screens of the thymus gland's protective mechanisms. Food is brought inside for examination to see if the body wants it, to see if the cells of the body will accept this matter and energy and utilize it for necessary purposes. It is very important to understand that the colon has a nasty job; it has to deal with those materials inside it that the body has decided are its enemies.

Emotion: Hate

Individuals who complained of colon problems also had a difficult time being rejected, or were in a constant state of rejection. This emotion increases in crescendo to what humankind considers the most violent rejection of all: hatred. Hate is a handy mechanism for separating yourself from another's energy field.

Hatred, at number 3, and love at number 2 can be further explained in this manner: Love allows another person to come in past the gates; it is taking a chance.

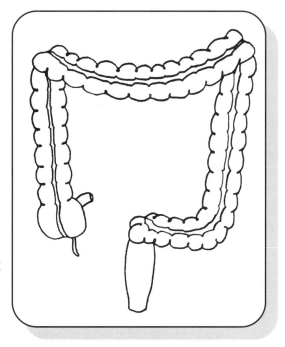

The Colon

81

When your partner gets inside to your basic mechanisms, that partner, if love has been mistaken for something else, can create absolute terror and havoc. This happens to many people who are "in love" and then find that they are in love with a person who doesn't really care for them. In such a case, the partner can actually rip the lover apart because he or she has been allowed inside.

If a person has a definite feeling of hate, he is rejecting or pushing away the idea that another person can even come near him. Therefore, there is no energy intersection and no "partner-energy" can be pushed undetected into the body. However, it must be understood that to hate someone, a person must have had <u>some</u> kind of intersection with him in the first place. Another's energies have been consumed in some fashion; much like foods must be consumed first, then analyzed and utilized. A human being attempts to emotionally accept another individual's ideas and plans and then tries to digest them. It is only after he realizes that the other individual's ideas and plans are poisons to his own system that he decides to reject them. The process of hatred comes about by the fact that the individual, once he has accepted or loved, cannot easily reject another person and his/her plans or ideas.

The real problem in hatred is that the individual is not able to properly get rid of the other offending, intersecting energy. This is how love/hate relationships build up. A person has allowed an individual to come into his life and intersect with his energies and now he can't get rid of him or her. The problem of not being able to reject happily and easily causes a buildup of hatred. It is the action of energies trying to get out of the system and not being able to that builds up the pressure-hatred situation. The individual's energies are jammed, resulting in hatred. The poisons within his system can't be released, so they're stuck inside him and he has to push them out as hard as he can. The pressure builds and builds and so does the hatred.

Condition: Detoxify

Mentally and spiritually, we must be able to rid ourselves of the condition of toxicity because this is causing a loss of energy. A person begins to hate because he is losing energy, time and motion; his abilities are dropping. He feels himself being taken away, his space dwindling. Someone is encroaching on his space and he can't get him or her out; he's trying to detoxify, but can't. He is trying to get the other person away from his energy fields so he can operate properly, but herein lies the problem: he is having a difficult time getting rid of this individual. If the number 3 comes up in the front of an analytical chain from a questionnaire or while scanning a person on the SAF infrared programs, we see that the SAFent once cared for someone or something and is now trying desperately to get out of the situation. It is very important to see this number 3 in this context, for it affects physical situations as well.

Mental Aspects

Mentally, with a 3, the person is poisoned. He can't see. His mind is jammed up and he can't think straight. A person with hatred has a narrow viewpoint. He can't see the world; he only looks through a tiny tube. He can't see the outside. He is trying to wash himself clean, but feels that inside there is an indelible print on his mind that will never go away.

Physical Aspects

An interesting correlation found throughout the years of reading chains of numbers and looking at different processes is that many individuals trapped in a condition of hatred are also constipated. They have an irregularity about them, and are unable to release toxins or poisons. Even an individual who complains of diarrhea exhibits a marked inability to "let go of things." His energies are snarled up as if someone had put a hook into him. The fishhook is in his mind. Something has happened and he's not able to get rid of it. He can't forget it; he can't let go. His physical state mimics his mental state. He is jammed up; he is not fluid, not regular, or not able to be synchronized. He has lost the ability to have any kind of regularity.

> *Mind energy, in connection with spiritual energy, produces a magnetic and electric attraction for toxins and traumas in the environment. There is a behavioral pattern that acts like an antenna and pulls these in to the body.*

4

Stomach

AT A GLANCE:
Emotion: Happy
Condition: Digestion

The stomach is assigned the number 4 in the SAF sequence. The stomach is the vessel of digestion; as such it may be considered the battleground for energies coming into the system that need to be converted. The ingestion of foodstuffs from the environment requires that there be some area designated as a conversion place. Any substance or entity coming into the body must have its mind changed; its purposes must be changed to suit the body's total plan. If this is not accomplished, then the substance will ultimately do it harm. The stomach is equipped with glands that secrete gastric juices and that are necessary to break down a food substance into chyme so it is ready for further digestion. The genetic blueprint of the human body directs these acids, fluids and chemicals; this in turn depends on the genetic ancestry of that person to provide the right materials necessary for dissolution of the entities that have been ingested. For example, if a person swallows glass, there is normally no blueprint in the system for the digestion of this substance. However, there have been some human beings that have developed an ability to decipher, break down with chemical codes and digest any foreign substance, even glass.

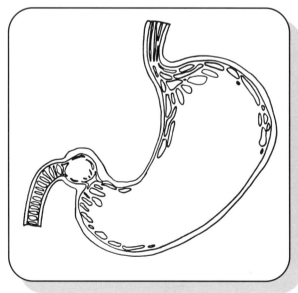

The Stomach

Emotion: Happy

Research has shown those individuals with stomach troubles invariably complained about unhappiness. Many ideas of existence correlate happiness to the stomach. When a person has a "full belly" he is happy. Happy actions exude from the stomach. A "good belly laugh" indicates that an individual is on his way to sheer happiness. The constitution of the United States guarantees that we the people are entitled to "the pursuit of happiness" (though not the attainment of it!) It would seem that if we were to desire complete and utter happiness, we would have to come up with a regimen so our system could digest anything.

Condition: Digestion

Digestion, of course, is the process whereby food is broken down mechanically and chemically so that it can be absorbed and used for cell metabolism. In many cases the term digestion transcends the physical sense. A person must be able to take apart <u>any energy or substance</u> that comes into his system. If an SAF Monitor finds the number 4 appears first in a chain of numbers derived from SAF scans and programs, then he knows that the person whose chain it is, is unhappy, he is unable to digest the circumstances around him. This can be a <u>mass circumstance</u> such as food, <u>energy circumstance</u>, such as a pattern of motion in the environment, or <u>concept circumstance</u> such as a condition developing between the human being and his environment.

Mental Aspects

When looking intently at the idea of digestion from a mental point of view, it is noted that people who have stomach troubles also have the inability to digest concepts in the mind. In this case, another word for digestion would be "understanding." If someone swallows an idea that is too large, he must break it down into smaller and smaller pieces until he can understand and digest it.

If we attempt to understand a huge problem all at once, and are not successful, then the solution would be to split it down, divide it and conquer it. Problems must be broken into finer parts to understand fully the conceptual meanings.

It is exciting to note that the whole process of digestion has been embodied into the SAF method. SAF is a digestive mental process. SAF is successful because it takes the complex problem of an individual and breaks it down into smaller, finer pieces. SAF gives a person the steps necessary to gain the ability to sequentially understand his problem. SAF gives an individual enough observable cause and effect so that he is now able to grasp the full meaning of how he could have gotten into a certain predicament.

Not having a plan, formula or sequence for figuring out problems can be a problem in itself. Problems accumulate with such tremendous energy and power that they can surely overwhelm an individual. For example, if an individual is trying to understand the economic systems of the world, the troubles in the Middle East, or the concept of death, etc., he must go down a long research or philosophical path to come to a satisfactory resolution. A one-word or one sentence explanation won't suffice. Human beings think in sequences. They are sequential beings; they must see the step-by-step pattern in order to understand concepts.

Physical Aspects

Individuals who have the number 4 in their SAF chain sequences were found to have pains in their stomachs. Many developed severe toxic states.

If you can't physically digest, then you are setting yourself up for trouble throughout your system. Many disease states, such as gout, rheumatism, arthritis, diabetes, etc., are direct results of an inability to digest. With diabetes, the afflicted individual can't digest sugars properly. In gout and rheumatism, uric acid builds up and poisons the system because the individual is not able to process it properly.

Of all the systems in a human being, digestion is extremely important from the cellular level all the way up to the mental level. It may be the focal point of the SAF method itself that individuals must learn to either digest substances or reject them away from the body to keep them from intersecting with the most precious energy pods inside the DNA/RNA.

It is important to note at this point that consuming drugs and over-the-counter medicines only serve to thwart that digestive process, for some of these materials are completely indigestible. Recreational drugs, such as LSD, marijuana, mescaline, crack, speed, etc. are also indigestible. They are taken into the system and never come out again. Common pain relievers such as aspirin (salicylic acid, acetaminophen) take 10 years to be eliminated from the body. Such pain relievers tend to also shut off mental images, the very images we need to see clearly and understand. All the while these substances are lodged in the body, they will create as much havoc as they can.

As we study SAF, we embrace the idea of cleaning out the physical system. We must remember that anything that goes into the body can potentially get stuck inside. The only way to recover is with a good digestive process. The enzymes within the system, produced by genetic command, are a direct result of the thymus gland's ability to observe and to recommend action against certain entities in the body. Yet with the thymus gland being the weakest gland, and the DNA/RNA being fooled on a consistent basis by the outside environment, foreign substances are able to sneak inside the body and then be released. The author says fooled because there are drugs and chemicals used today that can disguise unwanted substances, such as occurs with chelation therapy. So we have to be extremely aware and careful about our ingestion of substances. At the same time, we have to realize that there are so many pollutants, toxins and radioactive beams coming from a myriad of sources – air, water and food – that it becomes impossible to consistently eliminate activity in and around these polluting substances.

The only real answer is to have a detecting system whereby the individual can sense or discover the presence of an offending substance and come up with a direct way of editing or removing this poison from the body. Fortunately, the SAF method has been built for modern man. It is a tool for future existence, and it is exciting to note that the SAF system understands this problem of digestion. It is a tracking system used primarily to hunt down and seek out the offending, polluting substances in the body and come up with programs and plans for their elimination.

5

nterior Pituitary

AT A GLANCE:
Emotion: Observant
Condition: Coordinate

The anterior pituitary is the frontal part of the master gland, the pituitary, which has the ability to direct the plans of the genetic mechanism throughout the entire body, including the thyroid, the gonads, the adrenal cortex and other endocrine glands. It acts as a monitor to make sure that all the genetic programming mechanisms are followed through. All of what a person is and looks like is directed by the anterior pituitary gland - qualities such as hair and eye color, size, shape and body weight. The anterior pituitary gland is designated number 5 in SAF programming.

Emotion: Observant

In evaluating people with the SAF protocol, those with number 5 in the most prominent position (first in the chain sequence) were found to have an inability to observe reality. They had distorted perceptions. If asked to pick up a banana, he or she might reach for an apple. They might also drop things they are holding. The emotional capabilities are on hold; this person is just watching. His feelings are frozen. The number 5 individual has an emotional situation that is locked up.

Condition: Coordination

Number 5 is closely associated with number 2 in that there is a definite need for synchronization, harmony, and coordination, but number 5 is more concerned with the idea of control. When number 5 comes up in first position in an SAF numeric chain, it indicates the individual is losing control. He has encountered situations beyond his grasp and he is unable to coordinate his activities against the outside encroaching problem. These people are found to have growing prob-

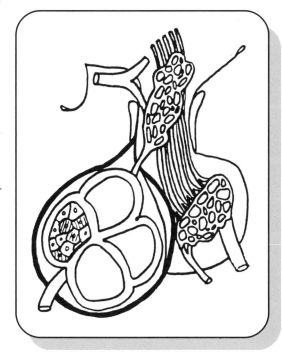

The Anterior Pituitary

lems about which they can't do anything. We find that many people in marital split ups where children are involved will show the number 5 in the first position on the chain. They can't control the situations that have been decided for them by judges and lawyers. They must work out visitation and monthly payments to their dislike and therefore are stuck having to do something over which they have absolutely no control. At one time or another most of us have encountered a number 5 situation; we have not been able to get a grip on our problems and steer ourselves back into control.

Mental Aspects

It seems that number 5 would embody the entire processing of SAF. It denotes an individual who has developed a slick kind of confusion that has earmarked him for trouble. As long as he can't dissolve or absorb the problem at hand, he will suffer. An individual must maintain mental control of his existence. He needs this control of his ideas and concepts to be certain that the necessary energies are present to complete them. For example, if an individual decided to build a garage, he must acquire the blueprints and the plans (the concept). Then he would need the money to buy all the materials and time to put them together (energy). Finally he would have to gather the timber, boards and nails (the mass). These things could be all present – concept, energy, and mass – but if an individual doesn't gain control of it, he may build a rickety garage, or not be able to complete the task at all.

The final culmination of our ability to control a situation is to build a perfect replica of what we had in mind. If we can't, we feel a subtle loss of control. It is the genetic promise that if an individual puts out an idea into his genetic programming mechanisms, that idea will appear in mass form. It is the wish-come-true mechanism that is part of the anterior pituitary complex and the fifth gland matrix in the SAF sequence. If we are not having our wishes come true, then we most certainly have a problem coordinating, and our ability to observe reality is locked up. We are not seeing things for what they really are and therefore we can't program our mind so that it will have a logical ending point.

This often happens to us when we are trying to develop relationships with other people. In the mental aspects of developing a human relationship with another person, it is often difficult to observe the attributes of another person that we like to copy and duplicate for a harmonious life together. Because of the necessary ability to lock in and harmonize in a loving way with another individual, number 5 is closely related to number 2. Number 5 embodies the idea of being able to control energies once they have intersected with our space. Once these energies are inside our system, if not controlled, they can wreck us. We don't need to develop a sense of trust for another human being, only the ability to observe and coolly control all circumstances that come into our own space. Even if the other person wanted to separate from or create other such mental traumas, we would be able to simply observe the situation and keep it under control. There are far too many people whose lives have been absolutely broken in half by the actions of another. This occurs dramatically because of the upsets of the anterior pituitary. If radiation from any source (including drugs, poisons or even a baseball bat smashing onto a person's head) is allowed to reach the anterior pituitary, the individual is in great danger. This master gland has to be in good working order not only for the physical ramifications of life, but also for the mental necessity of being able to solve problems and being able to see the exact reality, what IS.

Physical Aspects

Often a person who has a 5 up front in his chain will also wear glasses, hearing aids or some kind of assist for the senses. Persons having a distorted view will certainly need to have it corrected. Sometimes the distortion in the viewpoint of the individual is so great that it carries over into the sense machinery and affects vision. Light begins to curve and bend around them, and when they look at an apple, they might see a banana. So they really need to have a set of eyeglasses or some kind of visual assist. This is not a condemnation of individuals who wear sensory aids, but there can be some extreme examples that manifest.

When the anterior pituitary goes awry, subtle physical problems develop that are difficult to detect. The sinuses (chambers of gases) become affected. The anterior pituitary analyzes the gaseous state of the sinuses and takes apart the conditions, the actual specific gravity, the barometric pressure and the pressure sense of radiation around it. It is in this way that the thymus (1) and the anterior pituitary (5) work together in producing a perfect harmonic situation that is able to analyze the environment.

Number 5 in the first position of a chain might indicate the SAFent has a common cold. A common cold develops when a situation of high tension and energy is jammed into the system and affects the sinuses. The common cold, discussed in detail later, is a situation that is directly influenced by both halves of the pituitary gland – the posterior pituitary (21) and the anterior pituitary (5). The individual, at some point in time, suffered a loss and the anterior pituitary is trying to return or bring back the pressure to analyze that lost capability. The emotion of number 21 (the posterior pituitary) is grief or crying. When the sinuses are completely filled and there is drainage, the nose and eyes are running, the person is said to have a "cold." He is actually stifling a cry, a cry for help because something has been taken from him. We can see that these numbers work together to explain what the loss is about. Apparently, the tearing away of something from a human being creates an empty situation and tears at the control mechanisms, thus causing disharmony, which relates to the heart (2).

So, observation is essential. When reading the SAF chain of numbers, we gain a more accurate picture of what is being observed. The numbers are extremely important for you to be able to understand more about the physical, mental and spiritual aspects of yourself, your loved ones and the people you encounter every day.

6

iver

The liver, in SAF programming, is considered the fuse box and the battery. It is the electric power pack of an individual; within the liver are stored all the transcriptions and patterns of energy necessary for life. The combination of the anterior pituitary (5) with the liver (6) indicates an ability to coordinate activities and bring about necessary actions for life-sustaining survival in the environment.

The liver is found to be the sixth weakest organ due to its delicate electrical circuits connected to relationships with other human beings and the environment. For example, everyone contacted on a physical level, who has been very close to you (a mother, spouse, or anyone who has exchanged body fluids with you), will have a recording of this experience in the liver. The liver takes in all fluids or substances from another human being. The liver can be equated to a complex factory. It possesses all the tools for taking apart, breaking down and digesting the toxins and poisons that come into the system. It stores and filters the blood, secretes bile and converts sugar into glycogen.

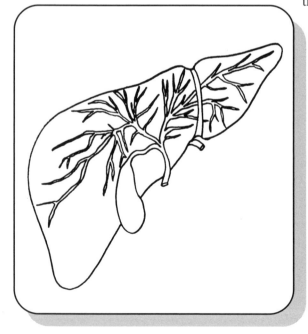

The Liver

4-6

When the liver (6) and the stomach (4) are linked together in the front of an SAF chain, this means that the individual has acquired what is called "civilization disease." In this instance, too many recordings are coming into his system that can't be fully digested, so he gets indigestion. Put 4 and 6 together and the person has biliousness, gas and rumbling in the stomach; the lower half of the body is making an incredible amount of noise trying to relocate and shuffle around all these toxins and materials that need to be tagged and bagged.

Emotion: Sadness

It has been found that when the number 6 (the liver) appeared first in the SAF chain, it was attached to the emotion of sadness.

Sadness is the opposite of happiness. It is a statement that the individual is "not happening." Unhappy means things are not going the way we want them to go, there is a break-up or a split-up, or there are situations in the environment intersecting with our energy. It is extremely important to note when a person has something or someone directly intersecting with his energy. Number 6 in a prominent place in the chain means that the liver is the area of this intersection.

The liver is the power pack and the home grounding structure; it is like the fuse box in the basement. If something from the environment, such as an infection, disease, toxin or even a mental upset comes in from the environment and intersects with that electrical circuitry, the person has a short circuit and blows a fuse. With the idea of sadness, we must immediately get the idea of a break. There is a disconnecting short circuit, and with the short circuit there is a problem with concept, energy and mass coordination. In such a case, the individual has an idea, may have the energy to complete the idea, and he puts much energy into completing the idea, but that idea doesn't come to fruition.

For example, a man desires to marry a certain woman. He courts her and spends lots of money on dinners, dates, jewelry, and furs and then is crushed when she runs off and marries someone else. His reaction is sadness. He has a broken feeling, much like a circuit that has been broken. In the English language, the word "liver" contains the word "live." When broken, the individual becomes aged and stops living.

The melancholia that occurs literally means "black bile." It turns black for a specific reason: blackness and darkness are the unknown. When a person's circuit is broken, there is an unknown wedge that prevents the individual from knowing the outcome.

Certainly the individual in the example would not have spent all his energy on the idea of marriage with no hope of realization. He should have foreseen what was going to happen. If his plan had been correct, he would have gotten what he wanted, but obviously his idea was not in the light. It was in the dark. There was information missing and he was gambling on mystery. He was hoping to create a situation that would be beneficial.

In the SAF method, then, what we attempt to do is take as much dark light, or what is called "black body light" and intersect it with the awareness of an individual and turn it into "white body light."

White body light is the information or energy that is known or conscious, and black body light is the information or energy that is unconscious or unknown. When something intersects with a white body light and turns it into black body light, the individual gets a broken, sad feeling. The differences between white body light and black body light will be studied thoroughly in this text because it is the nature of the SAF program to dissect and understand all the mysterious and invisible energies that surround a human being.

> *White body light is the information or energy that is known or conscious. Black body light is the information or energy that is unknown or unconscious. SAF links the two, shining a light into the darkness.*

Condition: Transmutation

The transmutation or changing of energies is the job of the liver; in the human being it is the system that helps him make all the proper changes throughout his life, for energy is constantly changing. As the earth tilts and orbits the sun, the seasons change; an individual's molecular and chemical structure must change or he will die. It is as simple as that. The poisons in the environment and the toxins that enter the system necessitate the change.

If number 6 comes up in front of the SAF chain, then we know that the SAFent's ability to change and redesign have been thwarted; there is a break somewhere that needs to be repaired. Number 6 is the number for keeping pace with changes. The saying "When in Rome, do as the Romans do," admonishes a person to keep pace with his environment or it will leave him behind in the dust. (It originally meant travelers to Rome must learn the way of the Romans, specifically to drink a lot of wine, which has definite effects on the liver!)

Mental Aspects

Mentally, an individual must be fast enough to keep pace with energy changes in the environment. If he is not quick enough in his intelligence and understanding, his perception of white body light is lacking and he will sink into the murk of black body light. There he will find much sadness.

If a person believes in hell and purgatory, he will find them on earth; they exist as the unsolved energy created in the mind. The pain and suffering of individuals who spend their time in hellish places comes about because the energy and mass build up to create situations of pressurized black body light. This crushes the person, thwarting his every activity. Even in mythology, the gods themselves were tortured because of their inability to understand and turn black body light into white body light situations.

Physical Aspects

The liver is a very important organ for the operation of the human mechanism. If it becomes disturbed in any way, the person will have a yellowish tinge to his appearance, called jaundice. Liver troubles greatly affect the eyesight, and, in this case tax the anterior pituitary (5) because the individual's perception has become distorted.

5-6

If your plans, programs, ideas, wishes, desires or dreams are being thwarted continually or even on a occasional basis; if black body light is intersecting with or taking over your white body light; if your mysterious half is becoming greater than your known half; or if you are more unconscious than you are conscious, then you are certainly unable to observe actual conditions. In this way, the liver (6) can disturb the anterior pituitary (5).

Errors in perception will naturally occur in people who are consistently taking recreational drugs, over-the-counter or prescription medicines; these toxins take away our ability to see things properly. Drugs rarely assist in anything except to override the action of some other poison. They are poisons fighting poisons, and the human body becomes a scorched battleground.

4-5-20

With liver upsets, digestive capability is greatly reduced. This would involve the stomach (4) and also the pancreas (20). When these numbers are in close proximity in a numerical chain, we know the SAFent may be having trouble digesting particles of life and living, as well as particles of food.

"It's better to light a candle than to curse the dark."

—Eleanor Roosevelt

7

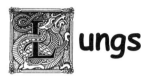

ungs

The lungs are in the seventh position; they consist of fibers and tissues of a relatively sensitive nature. Their matrix is used to deal with invisible gases, particularly oxygen and carbon dioxide. A lung respirator, used to take energies in from the outside, is nothing more than a gaseous digester machine.

Again, looking at the aspects of the body's operation, the lungs allow outside energies to intersect with its own systems. It takes them apart, dissects them, dissolves them, puts them into solution and then casts out the refuse the same way as the colon. The colon, however, deals with digesting masses while the lungs are an energy-digesting machine.

The lungs, of course, are essential for survival because of the constant need for oxygen digestion. Their purpose is respiration and aeration of the blood. We need continual intake. If we look at breathing as a type of digestion, we would see that we are constantly digesting gasses. By letting air into the system, it is necessary to make certain that the toxins and poisons, which are taken in along with the air, are processed <u>out</u> as rapidly as possible. Most of the trouble that arises with the lungs is created when toxins become lodged in the bronchi and then work their way through the bloodstream and into the cells and tissues where they take up root.

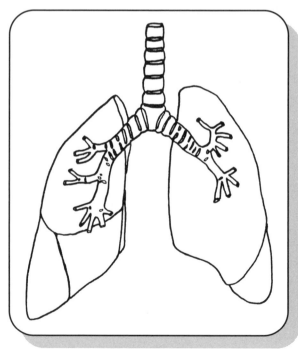

The Lungs

Emotion: Monotony

The emotion most closely depicted by SAFents found to have number 7 (the lungs) in the first position of their SAF chains is monotony. When we look at monotony, we see a chronic condition. In SAF programming, number 7 does not mean we are lucky. It means that whatever entity exists has been there for a long time. In SAF, 7 in association with any other organs or glands will point to this chronic situation.

5-7

For example, when the lungs (7) is connected with the anterior pituitary (5), it is indicative of what is called a common cough.

7-23

The common cough is a deep-set bronchial situation that can move into a condition of asthma that affects the lungs (7) and the spleen (23).

1-5-7

The lungs (7) also work with the thymus gland (1) and the anterior pituitary (5) to create a system of chronic exhaustion or tiredness. So we see that the appearance of number 7 gives us a continual monotonous voice. The SAFent may speak like a zombie. He may exude an idea that he is lost in some sort of deep miasma.

Condition: Vaporization

We have to watch number 7 because it is an energy number. It indicates dissolution and dispersion. It dissolves mass. It may not be the best condition to have when an individual is trying to create some matter, but it can be considered a lucky number when trying to explode or dissect some matter that has been chronic for a long period of time. We have to look at number 7 as the entity formed by the chronic condition itself. For example, if the SAFent has had a cold for two or three days and then it seems to go away, he must keep in mind that the cold is an entity and has an ability to create its own identity and a life of its own over a period of time. The cold symptoms are just 1/88 of the whole dragon, just the toe nail so to speak; the other 87/88 lies dormant inside the person. Usually, when a cold enters the system, it becomes a chronic condition.

Mental Aspects

The mental aspect of the lungs (7) is the notion of invisibility. If any body system confronts black body light more than others do, it would be the lungs, for the lungs operate wholly on a mass-less level. Certain entities are absorbed into the system that are invisible; the lungs, throughout their entire existence, are programmed to contend with invisible entities.

Physical Aspects

Human beings plagued with troubles of the lungs will find that this vital detoxification organ can affect every other organ in the body. The lungs are closely aligned with the kidneys (16), the skin (19) and the colon (3). In coordination with these organs the body efforts to process out all those elements that don't belong to it and absorb all the elements it wishes to keep. The confusions come when the emotional aspects intersect with the physical aspects. When an individual embodies a great deal of hatred (3) in his system, he certainly is unable to reject certain conditions around him, and these conditions may freeze up or become chronic problems on the skin (19). The factor of lungs (7) indicates that whatever problem is being worked on needs constant attention.

When noting 7 in the first position of the SAF chain, the SAFent may have trouble breathing. Breathing should be non-interesting and non-detectable. It should change to suit the amount of oxygen ingested and the amount of carbon dioxide rejected. However, if a person's breathing becomes labored or he is unable to correctly manage his circumstances, then he will have trouble.

7-24

If the lymph system (24) appears next to the lungs (7) in a chain, there is a good chance the individual is drawing in some toxicity from the air he is breathing. In many instances the person is either a smoker or is surrounded by people who smoke. This is indicated because 24 represents ingestion of drugs or toxins.

When the lungs are in proper working order, the body can be relatively healthy. If there is any trouble with the lungs whatsoever, the nail matrix and hair will begin to show signs of wear and tear.

7-19

If a person has number 7 in the first part of the chain, he will also have degradations of the skin (19) and other organs of the body. The skin (19) is important to observe when associated with the lungs (7) because the individual may have warts, moles, tumors, cysts, boils, pimples, acne or other signs that signal the inability of the lungs to reject toxins entering the system by way of the nose and mouth.

In other words, the lungs are having a difficult time processing out solid poisons coming in through the air, and therefore, the skin must take up the responsibility of trying to detoxify the entire system. When the skin fails, it is up to the kidneys (16) and the colon (3) to take up the slack. If they can't handle it, then the toxins and poisons wind up nestling in the colon (3), in the kidneys (16), or in the bones (9). If this occurs, then the individual is more prone to a cancerous situation. Remember that a human body tries to digest a substance or it tries to digest him. If a person has not been able to take apart a substance (digest=4), it may wind up in the most disadvantageous location possible. It could chew up some of the more vital processing areas such as the liver (6), heart (2) or the brain (12).

The number 7, because of its designation as chronic, can also indicate a possible hand-me-down genetic situation. In most cases when reading chains of numbers derived from human beings, ancient genetic conditions that may have lasted more than 100,000 years are indicated by the specific genetic changeover numbers 23-24. If a 7 is in the chain, it simply shows monotony, or a chronic condition. It means that for a long period of time, there was a constant exposure to a substance that may have had a detrimental effect. Whatever the condition may be, it must be addressed. Number 7 is vital to resolving the case because it gives the relative intensity of the physical, mental and spiritual situation. The number 7 in SAF chains intensifies any problem or condition.

> *"The more observation a SAFent makes of his own anchors, the more freedom he will experience."*

8

ex Organs

AT A GLANCE:
Emotion: Apathy
Condition: Reproduction

In the science of SAF, the sex organs are given the number 8. Included in this group are the male gonads and prostate gland, as well as the ovaries, uterus and mammary glands of the female.

Gamma rays and X-rays have an ability to atrophy and sterilize the sex organs.

Emotion: Apathy

Much controversy in the SAF program has been generated over why apathy correlates with the sex organs. Individuals who have had upsets involving the sex organs (such as herpes, AIDS, syphilis, gonorrhea, bacterial infections, yeast, candidiasis and many other non-specific infections and inflammations) also professed apathy. Included with the physical symptoms would be the mental disorders relating to these organs, including frigidity, sterility, impotence and many of the perverse sexual behaviors.

When the sex organs are disturbed by disease (mental or physical) there is a marked interference in the ability of the person to create. People who have had these conditions also complain of their inability to create, or to finish projects once started. Many SAFents who had sexual disturbances of one sort or another also expressed that long ago their projects, purposes or plans had been thwarted. When major creative cycles are thwarted, especially among writers, artists, painters and musicians, deep-set feelings of apathy ensue. An artist attempts to produce a work and present it to the public, but for some reason he is stymied or stalled or perhaps the public doesn't appreciate his creativity. This causes the artist to exhibit a low emotional state – apathy. In all cases where the number 8 is in the first position of the numerical chain, a state of apathy exists.

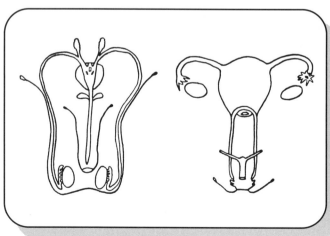

The Sex Organs

Condition: Reproduction

The number 8 embodies the entire knowledge of the disease entity and its existence in mankind. Diseases in any life form in existence (animal, vegetable, mineral, and other entities throughout all the solar systems, galaxies, and universes in space and time) have created a simple process whereby they reproduce. It is a necessary process, an extremely important one for the survival of any species or individual unit.

The action of one energy intersecting with another can be considered a sex act. The term "sex" in this sense is in actuality a misnomer, for the word sex means two divisions of organism, having characteristics of either male or female. It means to be different, or to be separated from another.

The fact is that sex indicates a difference and unsex indicates a unification. In this sense, when a mosquito inserts his long, narrow, proboscis into an individual's arm, he is not having sex, he is unsexing. The mosquito is trying to become part of the body and if he is successful, can withdraw more of the host's blood than he had in the first place. Unbeknownst to most individuals, this type of action is repeated billions upon billions of times per day.

To understand sex and to be aware of interconnecting your energy with the environment is to also understand that sex transcends the physical act. The point is that sex on a gross scale is a symbolic action, which represents the movements and activities of all energy throughout the day, throughout the entire life of the individual. In an electronic sense, words going into a tape recorder and then played back out may be considered a sex act. In a chemical sense, many molecules coming into a body and then being released in rhythmic fashion is a sex act - unification and then a release. The process of excretion from the colon and the bowels also could be likened to a sex act in the sense that materials are taken in and then, through peristalsis, are released.

Mental Aspects

On many fronts it is seen that in sexual activity there is also a power that comes from the mind. This sexual creativity comes from the ability of a person to intersect his ideas into other subjects or problems so that he can pull out the essential ideas and then can reproduce his own thoughts. The important quality affected when number 8 appears in a chain is the individual's ability to create.

When the number 8 is read with other numbers on an SAF chain, interesting data can be gleaned.

8-10

For instance, when sex organs (8) is found with the thyroid (10), it suggests that the SAFent is spending his energy unwisely.

8-11

If the sex organs (8) is next to veins and arteries (11) in a chain, it indicates that the individual is creating physical problems from mental worries.

8-17/18

When the sex organs (8) is found in connection with the endocrine system (17/18), it would show that the individual is losing his ability to create altogether; there is a cessation of productive ideas. The number 8 forms and combines with all the other numbers and aspects of SAF to create the mood and disposition of a person's creativity.

1-8

When a person is very aggressive about his ideas, poisonous with his concepts and aggressively tries to thwart or destroy another's plans, the sex organs (8) will be connected with the thymus (1). So if we see a 1-8 in an SAF chain, we know that the person is using energy in a negative way to hurt either himself or others.

8-12

If the combination were sex organs (8) with the brain (12), this would show that the individual is thinking of or wants to create an idea that is not yet fully formed in his mind. It indicates that ideas will be formed out of this parenthetical concept, 8-12.

In later chapters, more connections between numerical codes and their intersection with other numbers will be described. Attention is given to it here because the number 8 indicates excited actions between energies more than any other single number in SAF.

The number 8 represents the ability and the creativity to actually enhance the action of all other numbers, and of all other functions of chromosomal activity. This would include those that regulate detoxification and organization, those that are important for establishing location, and those that establish water balance in the body.

Physical Aspects

When the number 8 appears in the chain, the individual has difficulty with his entire system. The body is not able to create itself properly as has been blueprinted in its genes. This could involve upsets and degradation of the blood vessels in the body. The individual may find that his power is very low. His muscles may be lax. The most significant sign of upset is that the tone of the body is slack. The veins and arteries of the circulatory system may lack integrity. The writer will make no attempt to create a nomenclature for all the particular kinds of sexual disturbances and physical symptoms that accompany these organs. Suffice to say that any disturbance involving the sex organs and also any problem with the circulatory structure will be a primary indication that the number 8 is involved.

9

ones and Muscles

It is found in SAF programming that those individuals with the number 9 in the first position in the numerical chain will have some upset in the bone structures. The bones and muscles are weak in the presence of radiation, which in this case means not only nuclear effluence, but also background radiation from the sun, distant stars and other magnetic sources.

Emotion: Pain

The body's sensing mechanisms primarily interact among other structures to learn whether there are any encroaching entities in the vicinity. The body has its own early warning system, which can decipher when there is an invader present in the surround-ings, and at the same time, identify the exact type. This is made possible by the pain sensing mechanisms that work in coordination with the nervous system and other structures able to discern wavelength and frequency characteristics of energies that may enter the spaces of the body.

It may be most important to note that the factors providing the body with its sensing information on the pain level can be hyper-extended into unconsciousness, death and the zomboid level (the lowest level of human existence). A human being can sense activities occurring on a conscious level in the form of pain, but cannot knowingly track entities that are encroaching on the unconscious level. These unknown violations would include the actions of hypnosis, drugs, medications and similar programs. With the early warning sys-

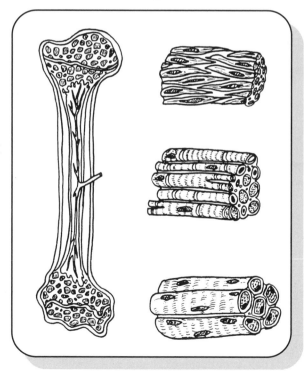

Bones and Muscles

tem and the SAF method, an individual can track all the sensing problems found in these lower strata.

Sensation and pain are polar opposites. Sensation tells the analytical intelligence of the human being (brain and mind) that we have lost something; it indicates energies are moving away from the body. They are being deleted. We are losing something. With pain, on the other hand, we gain something. It may be consciously or unconsciously acquired, wanted or unwanted. Pressures begin moving into body spaces and are violating the principle that two objects cannot occupy the same space at the same time.

Condition: Locomotion

Concerning this primary structure of the body, the skeletal system, number 9 relates to its movement. As with all energies and systems, if there is any impingement or encroachment from one group onto another, then there must be change, movement and space. The number 9 signifies this change, the ability to make moves from one space to another. This mechanism makes the actions of invasion, eating and parasite infestation possible. If one entity can't move on another, or doesn't have the locomotive power to change his location, then he certainly will not be able to invade.

When we notice the number 9 in the first number in the SAF numerical chain, it indicates that there are poisons present in the system. One specific designation for number 9 is rheumatism because, with this condition, poisons moving through the body are changing locations. However, it is not the fact that the poisons have just changed locations but that they have gotten into the body in the first place that is of paramount importance.

When number 9 appears, the system is showing that it has gained something it doesn't want. It has reached a new superior state of toxicity that it did not own before and it must find a way to detoxify (the colon, 3).

Mental Aspects

The ninth development of awareness intrinsic to the structure of any being is the needed ability to change mental position and to change viewpoint. As we move through daily life sequences, 9 is designated as the mental aspect that tracks our power to change our life toward the direction of peak performance. The SAF method arranges and organizes our action like no other program. The number 9 is extremely important because it gives us an ability to prioritize. SAF makes vital lists; lists of creative situations that trouble us. This allows us to invest all our energy into the most important actions first and the less important actions later. SAF also gives us the ability to arrange our choice of healing actions on a step-by-step scale of activity and achievement.

For example, if we were learning to swim, we would start by practicing the pre-basics, such as ducking our head under water. Much later our skills would improve and we may be able to perform various strokes. There is a specific sequencing arrangement that gives us the ability to accomplish easier tasks first and then harder tasks second, and so forth, until we are able to reach the expert level.

When number 9 appears as the first number in a chain, it indicates this person has an inability to prioritize, or to put events into a sequential order. It might be difficult to create organized situations out of chaos. He is not able to straighten confusions and put in order the organic and inorganic messes of his life. This suggests that toxins, poisons and diseases infesting his system are more regimented and organized than he is. He may not have the ordered aspect of mind to create structured activity in body, in mind and in spirit. He needs SAF programming to help him understand the basics of the step-by-step approach.

Physical Aspects

The most physical number of all is 9. The SAFent may be in pain, a physical reflex warning action of great importance. The ability to decipher and evaluate these warning signals differentiates a human being from an animal.

It should be noted that if you are prone to accidents or have continued collisions in the environment then 9 indicates troubles on a much deeper level. You may be unable to decipher the warnings of earlier pain profiles. Pain is always the alarm signal for the encroachment of a minor or major disease characteristic. It means you may be falling into some potentially dangerous pattern that could do you great harm or even kill you in the future.

If you find yourself in a situation where you have lost the ability to extricate yourself from problems and poisonous conditions, then you have probably ignored some primary pain reflex signal early in your life. For example, if a person were to suddenly find a cancerous condition, it is certainly not the result of traumas that have occurred in the last few months. He must have been ignoring or not understanding pain signals earlier in his life. In the incredibly chaotic mess created by civilization today, it is nearly impossible for individuals to decipher pain signals. Toxins and poisons released into the atmosphere are extremely complicated and cause bizarre energy signal patterns that inflict the body with pain that is difficult to process.

10

Thyroid

AT A GLANCE:
Emotion: Anxiety
Condition: Metabolization

The word thyroid, from the Greek *thyreos,* (large shield), and *eidos* (form) means a physical shield. Whereas the thymus (1) is the electronic invisible shield, the thyroid (10) is the shield for the physical form, the body. As such, the thyroid is a sentry to prevent toxins, poisons and other energies not belonging in the body to be processed out and kept away. Those people living in close proximity to nuclear power plants are slated to receive free potassium iodide to protect their thyroids and lower glands should a disaster occur. The thyroid also helps the anterior pituitary (5) regulate the appearance of the structure of the body.

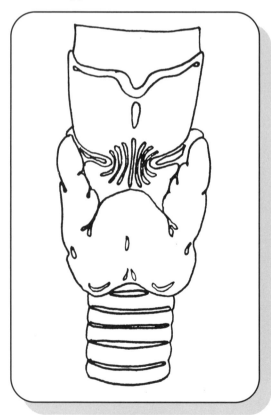

The Thyroid

Emotion: Anxiety

The emotion anxiety results when a person attempts to perceive what might happen in the future. Anxiety is generated because you have created some scenario in the past that is rickety and unsure at best, and you are holding that in place in the present. You might be worried that the plans and programs you have produced have not been powerful enough to sustain you throughout the interference of energies in the environment. Individuals who understand the mechanisms of survival will see that the thyroid is an intrinsic cog in the program of Life Energy and the ramifications of toxicity.

The thyroid can become very toxic and create a sensation of anxiety. A state of delirium tremens following drug or alcohol withdrawal is characteristic of thyroid upset. In this situation the thyroid becomes heavily toxic in its war against these pollutants, and causes a trembling sensation.

The thyroid is working hard to shake loose poison and move it from the system. It assists the transfer of toxins to the thymus (1) for final extraction. But when these two glands (the thymus and the thyroid) get together and are not successful, the individual is prone to body tumors. Goiter is a primary example of this condition.

Condition: Metabolization

The important consideration of the thyroid, in a conditional sense, is its ability to change the features of the body. The genetic blueprints, using the command centers of the anterior pituitary, affect the thyroid and will it to make its changes. In effect, the thyroid becomes the foreman of the body. It works in conjunction with the liver (6) to repair the body and to change its structure depending on the directives from the anterior pituitary.

Interference to the gene plans and programs are what give individuals the characteristic lumps, bumps and misshapen parts that are the cataloged anomalies of mankind. To give names to each one of these disease characteristics is really not necessary. The point is that an afflicted person has toxins and poisons that have worked their way into his system. These poisons will affect various organs. The SAF breakthrough is the development of a method that can detect the precise order in which these organs will be affected.

Heat, pressure and the variation of toxic influence will create a prioritizing sequence of invasion within the body. In other words, a disease condition has a target plan and zooms in on some areas of the organism for immediate invasion, while other areas are the targets for light invasions or remote invasions.

SAF can track all these disease characteristics because it understands these sequences. The point is, the thyroid has the ability to sense and pick up heat changes in the body, and in a very real way is the body's own infrared sensor. It is curious that when the thyroid is malfunctioning, the individual has a difficult time withstanding heat in the environment and heat changes in the body. When the thyroid feels the pressure from the heat changes, the person will receive erroneous signals concerning excess disease in the system. So the thyroid readings becoming extremely important as an assist to the SAF program.

Mental Aspects

Mentally we must learn to make changes in viewpoint. As was seen in the mental and physical aspects concerning the bones and muscles (9), we know that changes of time and space will affect the primary sequencing pattern. The thyroid has the important ability to foresee and carefully supervise these specific changes. The mental aspects of the thyroid gland must be able to withstand change; it is the most important and most necessary function of all activities.

An individual in excellent shape is able to change his mind and position with whatever circumstances arise. Conversely, if a person is ill and his thyroid is malfunctioning, then mentally he will be very rigid and his ideas will be stuck together.

10-15

When the thyroid (10) is connected with the hypothalamus and senses (15) then we have what is called a mental mass or a block. It has been found that writers who become stuck when attempting to write novels or technical data will exhibit a 10 and 15 in the foremost part of their numerical chains because mental masses are building up.

10-11

In the case where the thyroid (10) and the veins and arteries (11) become associated, it indicates that the individual has an inability to put his plans, dreams, desires and wishes into action. When (10) and (11) are seen together in a chain it means that there are peculiar upsets blocking the person's ability to be creative.

8-10

As was stated earlier, when the sex organs (8) and the thyroid (10) are associated, then the individual is wasting energy. He is not utilizing his potential to the fullest.

4-10

One of the most important aspects of the thyroid in the mental sense is its connection with the person's ability to digest ideas and concepts properly. When the stomach (4) and the thyroid (10) become coupled in a numerical chain, then the SAFent will be found to have difficulties controlling his emotional responses to people around him. There are many other connections for the number 10 on the mental aspects to be covered later in the text.

Physical Aspects

2-10

One of the most important physical aspects that is found with the thyroid (10) is its connection with the heart (2). When 2 and 10 are found in the same numerical chain, they denote rudimentary considerations for the viewing of the individual's condition. The link 2-10 indicates the extent of the person's inability to withstand insult and injury from the environment. This is the kind of insult, injury, break up, separation and loss that may physically damage the individual. It can tear at his heart and create disease there.

10-22

The thyroid certainly controls a lot of the physical aspects of the individual and must be considered in all programs used. When the thyroid (10) and the parathyroid (22) appear in a chain together, the individual is prone to spinal misalignment. He may have rickets, sciatica or spinal decay. It is extremely important for an SAF Monitor to spot 10-22 in any numeric sequence because these numbers suggest structural problems, and depending on their location in the chain, may indicate problems of long duration.

10-17/18

When the individual's thyroid is malfunctioning, he may become overweight. This is further indicated by the combination of thyroid (10) and endocrine system (17/18).

10-12

The number 10 combines with many other numbers in sequence chains to describe other physical and mental aspects such as the person's ability to change viewpoint and to understand new things in the environment. For example, an important rudimentary mental upset is the thyroid (10) and the brain (12) connection. In this case, we are primarily looking at a misunderstood situation, idea, concept or just overall confusion in the person's life. A 10-12 always indicates that the individual is having difficulty perceiving the true circumstances around him or understanding new concepts. This trouble may transcend into the physical sense when the person has the misfortune of translating the confusion into his body. Many of the pains and sensations, the odd feelings that he or she is just "not okay," energy exhaustion and all the poisons associated with modern-day living form a 10-12 phenomenon. It shows a basic confusion about how to behave to insure survival.

Number 10 is one of the most important in the SAF program because of its ability to monitor radiation in the system and because it can coordinate actions in a physical as well as a mental sense to achieve the genetic program of the body.

> *A thorough understanding of the SAF numbering system is the only thing that is essential for you to increase your self knowledge.*

11

Veins and

Arteries

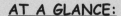

AT A GLANCE:
Emotion: Resentment
Condition: Circulation

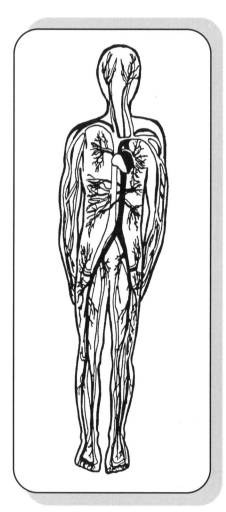

The veins and arteries of the lower extremities are considered an extension of the heart. This system is important in the respiration or the reflex echo pumping of the heart mechanism. Therefore, this system, designated number 11, should be monitored very closely.

Emotion: Resentment

When there is an 11 on the left side of an SAF chain, it indicates that actions taken by this person are causing deep-seated resentment. With resentment, an individual harbors ill feelings about some occurrence in the past. Such a person has continual upsets and attracts the same type of trauma over and over again. He dwells so much on these problems that they chronically draw more of the same to him.

Condition: Circulation

Those who have exhibited upsets involving the veins and arteries (11) have also complained of continual circulatory problems. The presence of 11 in an SAF chain indicates a chronic condition.

Mental Aspects

A person who has complained of being scattered or dispersed will always exhibit the number 11 in his chains. Such an individual must be careful not to be suffocated by holding onto the poisons in his mind for

Veins and Arteries of
the lower extremities

any long duration. However, he does not have traumas buried deep within his system beyond conscious reach. The person who carries on with an 11 is very cognizant of his traumatic experiences and puts a great deal of energy into this problem. He is constantly dwelling on the past. He is quite sure that the past problem he is focusing on is the source of all his troubles, when in reality there is something buried deep in his system of which he is <u>not</u> aware.

The term that could be used for an individual who exhibits an 11 is "scatterbrained." He puts much of his energy into other people's problems and troubles. He is a sensitive person who systematically absorbs problems from surrounding individuals. If his family or friends tell him a problem, <u>he</u> will worry about it for them.

11-14

When the veins and arteries of the lower extremities (11) connect with the mind (14), the individual may suffer tremendously because it increases his worry deficit. He is spending too much time trying to decipher problems that are not his own.

Physical Aspects

10-11

Often an individual with an 11 in his chain will show a predisposition to arteriosclerosis as a result of circulatory system degradation, especially when 10 (thyroid) is in the same chain. The integrity of the blood vessels is lost.

8-11

When the sex organs (8) are involved with the veins and arteries of the lower extremities (11), the individual will be found to have severely compromised his ability to maintain his muscle tone. He may exhibit a fresh crop of varicose veins or hemorrhoids. He may complain of constant pains in the arteries, such as those exhibited by patients who have phlebitis. The most important action for a person in this physical situation is to use chelating elements to detoxify the entire bloodstream as well as clean the fibers and walls of the veins and arteries. Such an individual is in great jeopardy because he is liable to develop poisonous situations in the soft tissues and more prone to cardiovascular and cerebro-vascular accidents (stroke).

11-14

The danger of stroke is especially great when the veins and arteries (11) are in connection with the mind (14) and the individual has what is termed "bursting headaches" or constant headaches. These are usually a warning signal of an impending stroke.

11-15

When the veins and arteries of the lower extremities (11) combine with the hypothalamus and the senses (15), the individual is creating tendencies in the body to harden vital organ structures. He must be very careful not to fall into this pattern.

11-16

This vital organ hardening occurs particularly in the kidney tubules when the veins and arteries of the lower extremities (11) are in combination with the kidneys (16) in an SAF chain.

11- any number

Of course, when 11 is connected with any number, the combination pinpoints the specific area in which there is a breakdown of circulation, either the inhibition of circulation, or the action of total dispersal. The dispersion problem is included primarily under mental aspects, whereas the solidification problems relate more to the physical aspects of the body.

> *"The more of the unconscious we are capable of making conscious, the more of life we integrate." — Carl Jung*

12

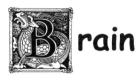rain

The brain, the central nervous system control factor, is considered the main operation base. Because SAF is based on physical electrical output, the laws of electricity, magnetism and radiational studies, the brain is a fitting position as the epicenter of the program. SAF is not physical, mental or spiritual alone, but a trinity of these three. The brain is that physical area that is the absolute core of operations for spirit energy, mind energy and physical energy. It is the meeting ground for SAF intellect and current everyday science; it is an area upon which both segments of philosophy can agree. The brain is the bridge between known and unknown information.

Emotion: Nervousness

The word nervous typifies the action of not only the brain but of the SAF program and its constituent parts, in that SAF has the capability of tapping into the nervous system and reading the electrical functions. SAF monitoring is accomplished by several methods. One way is with an infrared scan, perfected for analyzing the neurovascular reactions of the body. Just as effective, and in many ways preferred, is with the questionnaires (SAF-120 for physical symptoms or the Stress-120 for emotional symptoms), which are used to ascertain the current realizable symptomatology of any individual. Subjective symptomatology is very important, and is fostered by pain and sensation grids developed by the nervous system. These reactions cause symptoms that are brought to the attention of the person completing the SAF-120 or the Stress-120. It is because of the nervous system that

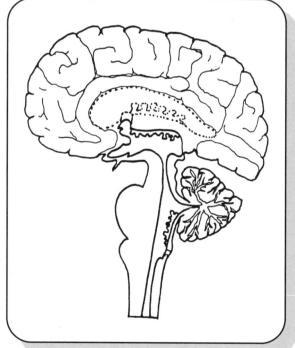

The Brain

SAF is capable of doing what it does. The SAF infrared scanning works primarily on a stimulus-response basis whereby energy can be monitored through relay areas such as the hands, the feet, the face and the entire organic system of the body.

The emotion of nervousness indicates there is unusual activity in the nervous system. This activity must be analyzed more closely to get a better idea of what is going on in the system to see if something extra is functioning there.

When you are nervous it means that your systems have been turned on, that something is happening, and those actions are occurring on a conscious as well as an unconscious level. We are vitally interested in understanding more about how the brain projects this energy, but at the same time we must analyze the patterns of nervous response in the whole body.

Condition: Electrification

The energy portals developed through the SAF grid work are important to the symptomatology of the system as they are patterned after the brain's own pathways. The word electrification indicates "a splitting apart" or a "segmenting." The SAF program is able to dissect (or split apart) and understand conglomerations of masses unreadable by human beings, which is also a purpose of the brain. All of the upset and confusions causing toxicity in the system are directly related to the brain's inability to segment and analyze confusions.

Confusions that are not dissected will well up into tremendous balls of mass that are dark and unreadable, so it is important to realize that a core idea of the program is to be able to split apart, dissect and thus understand. This is what the brain does when functioning properly.

SAF is the greatest problem-solving method to come along since the beginning of time. It can dissect simple problems as well as the most confusing complexities anyone could have. As a problem-solving machine, it eats problems consistently and willingly, and will do as much as its master commands. This is true if using any of the subjective questionnaires or the infrared sensor. No matter how many questions are constructed, the Self Awareness Formulas will perform to find the answers.

Mental Aspects

The mental aspects related to number 12 are directed toward the idea of unknown barriers, which are developed beyond the reach or understanding of the individual. Be aware that whenever a 12 appears in any SAF chain, there is attention positioned on the unknown. Nervousness occurs when an individual is not able to understand the unseen. There must be some unknown invisible quantity that is part of his problem, and yet he can't see it.

When developing a program for nervousness, we must look at the processing power of the individual, especially in coordination with other glands and organs.

10-12

If the thyroid (10) gets in close proximity to the brain (12) on a numerical chain, then the individual has misunderstandings and confusions present. These are rudimentary confusions that must be sorted out very quickly.

12-13

When the brain (12) is connected to the adrenal glands (13) in a chain, then the individual has many projects and plans left incomplete. His energy is scattered because bits of it remain focused on the unfinished projects; he might not be able to muster enough energy to complete his plans. In a physical sense, these unfinished projects may create a condition of insomnia, which may be detrimental. (See 12-13 sequences below).

Physical Aspects

Physical upsets involving the brain (12) are primarily headaches, neuralgia and nervousness. This nerve reaction, of course, may be due to mental conflicts 90% of the time but may also be part of a biochemical upset wherein the elements calcium and magnesium are out of balance.

12-17/18

When the brain (12) is associated with the endocrine system (17/18), the individual may exhibit signs of food allergies. He may be consuming something that is upsetting the biochemical balance of the body and therefore causing the condition of nervousness. This can be analyzed with the SAF system to develop an idea to which foods the person is allergic.

12-13

If the SAFent's chain connects the brain (12) and the adrenal glands (13), then there may be insomnia, the inability to sleep or gain rest. In this particular context, gaining rest comes not only from sleeping but also from getting REM sleep (Rapid Eye Movement), which is a dreaming state. REM sleep physically discharges electrical activity from the body and causes a deep relaxation. Often people feel they are getting enough rest because they "slept like a rock," but in reality, they are overshooting the REM state; therefore, they are not getting the much-needed physical release of electrical charge. This can cause varying upsets, such as daytime exhaustion or a specific type of nervous energy. This typifies the 12-13 individual.

12- with any other SAF number

The idea of number 12 in a chain of numbers bespeaks the concept of hidden energy. The organ found next to 12 would be the primary location of the upset: there is some unknown, hidden or obscure condition involved.

13

drenal Glands

AT A GLANCE:
Emotion: Courage
Condition: Capacitance

Designated number 13, the adrenal glands are located above the kidneys and are comprised of the cortex (produces steroid hormones) and the medulla (supplies epinephrine and norepinephrine.)

These glands are the spark plugs of the body, carrying enough power to give an individual 14 trillion volts of energy. If all the cells in the body were coordinated with the electric capacities of the adrenal glands, an individual would be able to pick up two locomotives, one in each hand. Indeed, we have all heard of heroic instances where the adrenal glands kicked in and made it possible for a slight person to lift a 2000-pound car to save a hurt loved one. The reason the adrenal glands don't seem to give us the capability of superhuman strength on an everyday basis is because of the checks and balances issued by the rest of the organs, especially the anterior pituitary and the gonads.

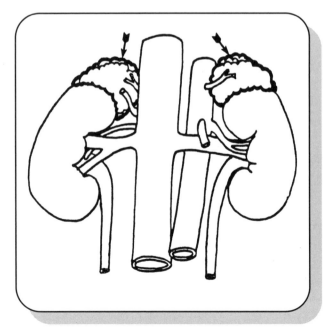

The Adrenal Glands

Emotion: Courage

The adrenal glands are the mechanism of courage in the body. Courage, in this sense, is the ability to put up with stress and defend against attack. In coordination with the thymus gland (1), the adrenal glands (13) are what gives us our base immunity system. They are extremely important in all phases of courage: physical, mental and spiritual. It is our ability to act with courage that elevates us above all other organic life.

No matter how much stress is put upon him, a courageous individual seems able to continue along the same course of action in his everyday life. Many times we don't realize we are in a courageous situation because the stress has mounted by increments without our awareness. Such people are fighting heroic battles day in and day out. We view courage as a feeling that occurs in the face of imminent, extreme and acute danger, but this is not always the case. Often we are exposed to chronic circumstances, which puts an inordinate amount of stress on our system, and causes us to need adrenal strength on a subconscious level. This could include the body's battle against allergies or viruses. Unfortunately, this type of courageous activity starves off the adrenal powers, diminishing our ability to cope with sudden danger at a future time.

Condition: Capacitance

The adrenal glands exemplify our ability to do work and to perform functions. It has been seen when the number 13 appears in an SAF numerical chain that the complaints included exhaustion and an inability to perform under any kind of stress.

13-16

Often the adrenal glands (13) will have a connection with the kidneys (16) in a chain sequence. This could be called the failed test of strength or courage, for 13 indicates the emotion courage while 16 indicates fear. The individual, at some time in the past, found himself in a position where he was on the horns of a dilemma; he had an opportunity to become a hero. Did he act and let his courage carry him through to completion, or did he run the other way? Many times when a 13-16 appears, it is indicative that the person has turned away in the face of danger.

13-17/18

Another interesting combination is the adrenals (13) coupled with the endocrine system (17/18). When viewing this set, it demonstrates that the individual feels a loss for the zest of living. This loss of desire to participate in life was caused by some severe trauma in the past that was powerful enough to drain the adrenal glands of their strength and energy. Indeed, upon questioning, this was found to be true.

As was seen in the earlier chapters of this book, we might have the illusion that our energy or power has been taken away from us; however, this is impossible, for the genetic storage memories are not erasable. They are always present. All that has occurred is that some trauma or energy has misaligned or blocked the pathways we normally use to retrieve this power from our genetic storage banks. So, the SAF sequence (13-17/18), shows that the trauma, whatever it was, was powerful enough to convince us we could not reach back into our energy banks. We could not have energy anymore.

The content of the trauma is a powerful mechanism that is affectionately labeled "The Dragon" in SAF training, and it is usually indicated by the numbers 17/18. When the dragon (the trauma) in our life is powerful enough to convince us there is no such thing as energy, then it can successfully thwart even the most powerful person in his ability to perform tasks. The important thing to remember is that these dragons exist in many different areas or sub-strata of energy within a person, so we could conceivably have energy in some areas and have none in others. This is what creates phobias and fears. We may have the ability to fly an airplane or drive a car yet have a distinct and terrible fear of elevators or crowds of people. This happens because this particular dragon (17/18) is powerful enough to jam our mental/physical circuitry and cause us to believe we have no power in these areas.

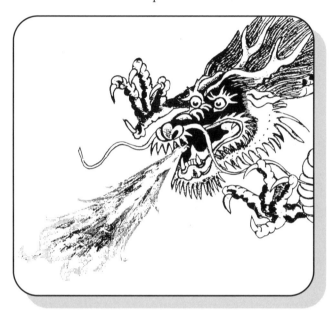

The content of the trauma is a powerful mechanism affectionately labeled "The Dragon" in SAF.

Mental Aspects

13-20

One of the most powerful mental viewpoints involving the adrenal glands (13), is its connection with the pancreas (20). This sequence relates to the inability of a person to cope with the loss of possessions or items, and especially locations such as their home. Those who have a 13-20 combination in the chain are often found to be homesick, but in many cases it is subconscious. Strange as it sounds, it is not uncommon for us to have a specific problem wherein some of our organs are "homesick" and others are not.

For example, if someone has lived for some time in rural Louisiana and then relocates to New York City's winter climate, a few of his body parts may still be functionally attuned to the bayou while the others have caught up with the new location. Examples of this phenomenon have been put to music. Remember the popular song, "I Left My Heart in San Francisco"? This lack of synchronization causes an outflanking of the energies or causes us to feel dispersed in our present surroundings. We may be exhausted or have hypoglycemia, a condition in which our energy rises and falls at certain intervals during the day. Particular hours of the day and specific events will cause a loss of energy. At the same time we may notice that we are losing muscular strength, and that the body is starting to drain itself of energy. This is because various organs are not in harmony or synchronization with the rest of the body and we are starting to lose our physical performance abilities. This would especially be true if the bones and muscles (9) were also present in the numerical sequence, (9-13-20).

13-14

When the adrenal glands (13) are closely connected with the mind (14), then the individual may complain of poor eyesight, astigmatism, myopia, or an inability to focus properly. This situation arises because the person is having trouble viewing reality. His mind is not able to face certain traumatic situations; therefore he has trouble seeing exactly what is real and what isn't real in the environment. Life images may become bent when they hit the plane of the body; actual images may become distorted.

Physical Aspects

Many physical problems involving the adrenal glands are very marked. A person may have bronzing of the skin, but more importantly, there is that factor of exhaustion. The person may be run down and unable to cope with stress. He may not be able to handle physical pressures or do as much physical work as before.

10-13

When the adrenal glands (13) are tied with the thyroid (10), the individual may be in the throes of some physical abnormalities causing him to have mal-absorption or trouble with his diet. It is indicative of a problem involving the acceptance and the rejection of foodstuffs. What he is eating may be causing allergic reactions. The force and the power of the adrenal glands initiate the fight against allergens, unwanted substances and toxins in the body, and this would especially be true if the thymus (1) and spleen (23) were also present in the chain, (1-10-13-23).

13-20

As mentioned in the mental aspects, when the adrenal glands (13) connect with the pancreas (20), the person exhibits, on a physical level, loss of muscular integrity. In other words, he may be cannibalizing his body by using his own protein structures more than usual for energy because there may be some renegade allergens such as a superoxide in the body.

12-13

Another physical factor for observation is the combination of the brain (12) and the adrenal glands (13). These numbers together are directly related to the action of the body trying to get rid of traumatic circumstances during the day.

As we go about our daily life, electric pressures from the environment in the form of mental pictures and experiences (22) are recorded in the bones and muscles (9). The logical sequence of events would be that the brain (12) and the adrenal glands (13) must be harmonized so that the body can reject the toxins of experience (22).

Some experiences (22) are pleasant (4) and some are unpleasant (6), but the residual charge that causes friction energy and develops into capacitance (13) must be eliminated.

Sleep is very necessary so we can discharge, deeply discharge, the spurious toxins of a normal day's activity. If we don't reach full REM sleep, we are not totally relieving our tired body and our weary mind of the infiltrating toxins that may become latent within our system. As each un-refreshed night goes by, the errant damaging electric charges in the body will remain charged. This then increases the chances that there will be more difficulty with simple pressures and mundane stress on a daily basis. If we don't reach the much-needed REM sleep, then we are constantly backing up electrical charges and unwanted friction energies that are strong enough to generate heat in any organ.

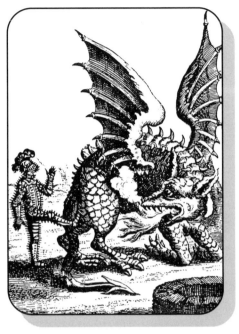

If we are able to discharge all toxins from our system, we will certainly be dragon-free for our whole life.

Many of the disease entities created by the aforementioned process will be depicted in the rest of this handbook. For now, you should know that dragons could be created by a combination of simple stresses that are picked up during daily life and refuse to be discharged from the body. It makes sense that if we are able to discharge all toxins from our system we will certainly be dragon-free for our whole life. It is interesting to note that when we successfully rest, we attain a state of alpha, which is the true wavelength or circumference of planet Earth. This gives us a proper grounding state and excitedly draws toxins and all unwanted electrical phenomenon, not associated with the body, back into the earth where they belong. If we could actually view this scene we would see dragons by the hundreds being pulled from the body toward the earth.

> *When an individual attains a state of alpha, dragons are pulled from his body toward the earth.*

14

ind

AT A GLANCE:
Emotion: Wonder
Condition: Analyzation

Probably the most mysterious part of a human being is his mind. Many philosophers, scientists and poets throughout the ages have tried to detect, dissect and explain the mind and its working parts. When groups of people are asked where the mind is located, we hear a variety of answers. Many are confused. They don't understand what a mind is. They think the mind is in the brain.

In the science of SAF, the mind is given the number 14. It is considered to be an electromagnetic aura that invades, infests and pervades every cell and nuclei of the body, especially by using command centers <u>around</u> the brain. In essence, the subject of our SAF work is the diligent and arduous study of the electroplasmic field, those various halos or auras that steadfastly revolve around every human being. The electroplasmic field is discussed in detail in *The Promethion.*

Paintings and mosaics from various periods in history have depicted saints and martyrs with very bright golden halos, for it was known that this golden aura showed the most harmony and balance of mental continuity. Human beings are not normally shown with halos because they have the basic but unfortunate problem of not knowing where their minds are located.

The mind appears to cup the brain and the skull, and therein stores numerous tiny microfine energies of various wavelengths. When speaking of wavelengths in the mind, we look at 1×10^{-30} (one times 10 to the negative 30th power) as a long wavelength, and 1×10^{-3000} (one times 10 to the negative 3,000th power) as a shorter wavelength.

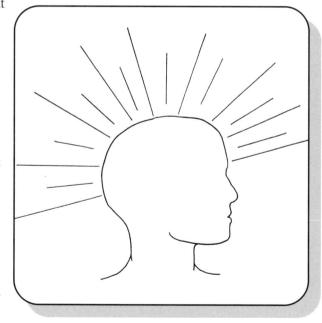

The Mind

The shorter wavelengths register the deep past. In the mind these will be connections we have to genetic philosophies handed down by our remote ancestry as present in the DNA/RNA. The longer wavelengths register a period closer to the present time. Many practitioners in the field of homeopathy become befuddled by the action of their high potency remedies. High potency homeopathic remedies have concentrations of incredible diminution, such as 1:1,000,000, that is one drop of substance to one million drops of water, a short wavelength. When taking high potency homeopathic remedies such as this, people may have the unfortunate reaction of having their ancestral memory files yanked out of their minds, ready to be examined by a practitioner who didn't know these were there in the first place!

It is crucial when doing SAF programming or <u>any</u> enlightenment procedure involving mental treks into the past that these past life wavelengths are in proper order by following the SAF method. If the short wavelength energies accidentally become longer, their power that existed in the past (even up to 500,000 years ago) can float into the present time and create havoc in a person's life. The wavelength of a past remembrance is brought forward from ancestral times when energy is pumped into it. This phenomenon can occur when homeopathic practitioners give their patients high potency remedies too often.

Many people don't even know they have these particular wavelengths and stored information so they certainly would never intentionally pump energy into them. People who dabble in past lives and other kinds of self-awareness routines that involve time travel may inadvertently be stoking the fires of a gargantuan dragon that lives in their past ancestry (the cell has all of this data recorded). It may be difficult to imagine before you have done SAF programming, that you can summarily be destroyed by actions of your ancestors that occurred 500,000 years ago. So it is imperative that the correct information is known, that all the programs are given properly, and that those programs produce the results desired by the individual.

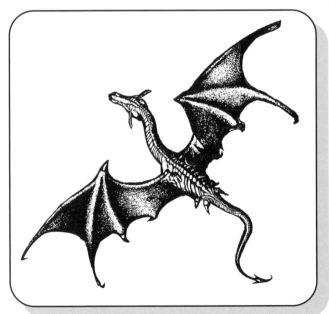

Dragons can float into present time and create havoc in a person's life.

When taking high potency homeopathic remedies too often, people may have the unfortunate reaction of having ancestral memories come to the surface.

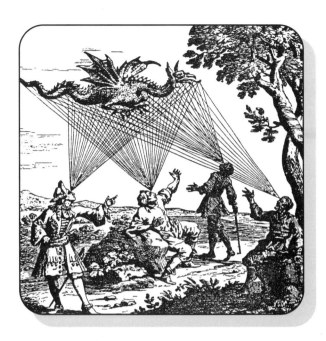

Emotion: Wonder

When SAFents produced numerical chains with the number 14 occupying the lead position, they had given a major complaint of chronic worry or mental disturbances.

The SAF program has been carefully developed to be sure that a person has a good understanding of the processes of the mind and the body. These special formulas cause the correct intersection of mind and body. The SAF philosophy embraces the concept that individuals can control an illness that may have a psychosomatic origin.

A person who consistently develops a 14 in an SAF chain must have his attention focused squarely on upsetting subjects. This person most likely lets his imagination run away with him. Depending upon which SAF format was used (questionnaire or infrared scan) the person may have a good deal of fantasy inter-playing with his problem. He may believe he has some particular condition when in reality he does not. Often when the number 14 shows up in the chain it is because an examining practitioner or family doctor has told the supplicating individual that he has had a certain harmful condition. When the number 14 is consistently present, there is a good chance the person may have been misdiagnosed. In such a situation, the hypothalamus (15), the anterior pituitary (5) and the lymph system (24) will be in close proximity with the mind (14).

SAF chains and 5-14-15-24 Combinations

1-2-<u>5</u>-<u>14</u>-<u>15</u>-<u>24</u>-16-17/18-3-9 ➤ wrong treatment currently

<u>5</u>-2-3-<u>14</u>-6-<u>15</u>-1-<u>24</u> ➤ drug poison in liver

<u>14</u>-16-8-<u>15</u>-<u>24</u>-6-7-<u>5</u>-10 ➤ drug causing delirium

20-21-<u>24</u>-<u>5</u>-4-<u>14</u>-17/18-<u>15</u> ➤ drug-induced hysteria

3-4-<u>5</u>-20-17/18-<u>15</u>-<u>24</u>-9-11-<u>14</u> ➤ psychosis caused by a drug

<u>15</u>-<u>5</u>-1-3-4-6-<u>14</u>-<u>24</u> ➤ misdiagnosis

<u>24</u>-1-3-6-<u>15</u>-4-<u>5</u>-17/18-<u>14</u> ➤ hallucination

1-<u>5</u>-<u>15</u>-12-13-<u>14</u>-2-<u>24</u> ➤ drug stupor

2-6-<u>24</u>-<u>15</u>-<u>14</u>-<u>5</u>-10-12 ➤ drug-induced coma

<u>14</u>-<u>24</u>-1-<u>5</u>-<u>15</u>-2-10-13 ➤ iatrogenic disease

We should be careful if the 14 is up front (to the left) in an SAF chain for it shows an active, powerful imagination process and, on the lighter side, the person may also be worried about the SAF test results! This is very possible, depending on how the SAF Monitor guides the SAFent through his or her program.

Condition: Analyzation

The number 14 designates worried persons who are constantly mentally computing and intensely pondering their troubles. The mind (14) doesn't represent the spirit; these are always separate, although there is a connection. A 14 appearing in the chain may represent a curious person with encircling worries and low self-esteem.

14-17/18

When the mind (14) is connected to the endocrine system (17/18) then we consider a very rudimentary problem, called general business troubles or environmental troubles. If the 14-17/18 combination has the sex organs (8) mirrored to it (14-X-X-8-X-X-17/18), then it is indicative of family troubles. If the 14-17/18 has the hypothalamus (15) near-by, then it is indicative of business troubles, specifically related to economics rather than family.

13-14

If the mind (14) is associated with the adrenal glands (13), the individual is having difficulty with his ability to accurately perceive his environment and his surroundings.

14-22

When the mind (14) is connected to the parathyroid (22), it indicates that the SAFent may be angry about situations. His dim confusions of the mind cause him to select wrong targets in his precarious environment. He may be picking on troubles that are really obsolete or are not of the right value. He may have altered erroneously what is important when considering a correct course of action. For example, if you are in dire need of a job and you are out shooting pool in the afternoon because you feel you need a career change, then you are making the wrong decisions.

The mind (14) in different combinations may appear anywhere and in any order on the SAF chain.

14-17/18-15	➤ business or financial troubles
14-17/18	➤ family difficulties
13-14	➤ perception
14-22	➤ angry, alters what is important
1-14	➤ psychic invasion
14-15	➤ insanity

Psychic or Mental Invasion (1-14)

A (11-<u>1</u>-20-<u>14</u>-23-24-5-6-7)

B (16-<u>14</u>-2-3-10-<u>1</u>)

In chain A, the condition is more acute, the 1-14 are close together in the chain.

In chain B, the condition is improving, demonstrated by the 1-14 numbers being more spread apart, reversed, and moving to the back (right) of the chain.

Mental Aspects

1-14

Because the number 14 is considered a mental phenomenon, it is important to note that when the thymus (1) is in connection with the mind (14), there exists a condition of mental or psychic invasion. The person is definitely afraid of random confrontations with other disoriented people because he can't put up with their sporadic impingement on his soul. His energies are not organized or powerful enough to ward off these hap-

123

hazard situations in the pressing environment, especially when in communication with other people.

14-15

When the mind (14) is connected with the hypothalamus (15), the individual is definitely showing patterns of distortion, mental derangement and temporary or continued stages of insanity. He has to make certain that his perceptions are accurate and precise if he wishes a chance at optimum survival.

Physical Aspects

The physical relationship of the body to the mind induces the psychosomatic condition. Because the mind is wired into the main impeller (a junction were physical matter, electricity and psychic power meet), the mind can easily cause the motor and sensory areas of the brain to function properly or improperly. The mind is able to create various situations that are of great importance to the mind and body on a demand basis. The mind has the ability, when under deep stress, to create violent physical reactions, one of the most powerful and injurious being a stroke.

10-11-14

When observing the mind (14) in an SAF chain, if it is connected with the veins and arteries of the lower extremities (11) and the veins and arteries of the upper extremities along with the thyroid (10), then the person should be wary that his mind is impinging information on the body that the body can't handle. He may be overtaxing the frail physical structure of the body with powerful energies that are too cogent for those specific cells. The number link 11-14 means we may be working on a condition of burnout. Different positions and combinations with surrounding numbers will further define the meaning.

SAF Chains and examples of 11-14

1-2-4-10-<u>11-14</u>-20-24-3-5 ➤ stroke

<u>11</u>-5-6-12-<u>14</u>-17/18-23 ➤ headache

22-<u>14</u>-1-3-5-<u>11</u> ➤ light pressure in head

3-22-<u>11</u>-6-7-8-9-<u>14</u>-21-24 ➤ headache worsening

5-7-16-<u>14</u>-21-9-3-<u>11</u>-2-4-10 ➤ headache getting better

<u>14</u>-17/18-15-21-3-22-16-<u>11</u> ➤ headache gone

<u>11</u>-12-13-15-16-17/18-2 -5-10-<u>14</u> ➤ headache potential

2-10-4-<u>11</u>-21-<u>14</u>-20-11 ➤ brain wave imbalance

<u>11-14</u>-22-2-10-15-4-21-5-6 ➤ loss of memory

14-17/18

When the mind (14) is connected with the endocrine system (17/18), then the person may be creating a definite scenario for building up fat cells in the body for protection from the overloads of business and family troubles coming from his immediate environment. The link 14-17/18 indicates a certain raunchy trauma from the deep past may be stealthily creeping into the unsuspecting wide-open mind portals and busily working on the delicate circuits therein. These traumas (dragons) are loaded with raw electrical charge just the way a murderous tornado or a wild electrical storm seethes and crackles with lightning. When a 14-17/18 comes up in a numerical chain, it may be indicating that the person could be in the throes of a maverick mental electrical storm; this is one of the primary sources for creation of psychosomatic illnesses.

"SAFents find that conventional ways of thinking do no good in the face of true dragons."

15

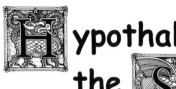 ypothalamus and the 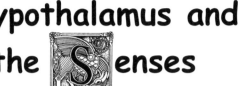 enses

AT A GLANCE:
Emotion: Attention
Condition: Evaluation

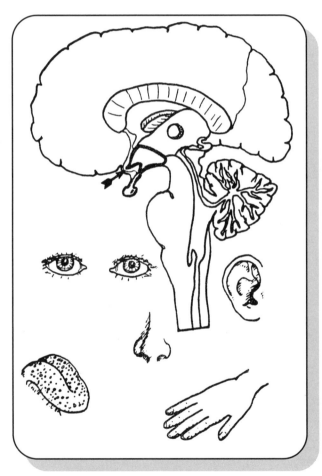

The Hypothalamus and the Senses

The hypothalamus (15) is directly associated with the complete balance of the human body and its deliberate daily functions as far as accurate regulation of heat and cold, appetite, and sex drive. This gland system activates and integrates the autonomic mechanisms and activities, endocrine and somatic functions. It controls the ability of the human being to discern stress and various patterns of pressure on each sense level. Therefore, in the science of SAF, the term hypothalamus (15) also incorporates the senses: seeing, hearing, smell, taste and touch, as well as the perception of time if the brain (12) is in the same numerical chain.

When the mind (14) is associated with the hypothalamus (15), then we think of sight. When the anterior pituitary (5) is in close proximity on a chain with the hypothalamus (15), then we consider hearing. When the lungs (7) are associated with the hypothalamus (15) in a chain, we are more interested in the activities of the sense of smell. When the stomach (4) is aligned with the hypothalamus (15) in a chain we consider the sense of taste. When the bones and muscles (9) are present along with the hypothalamus (15) in a sequence of numbers, we study the sense of touch.

4-15 ➤ taste
5-15 ➤ hearing
7-15 ➤ smell
9-15 ➤ touch
12-15 ➤ perception of time
14-15 ➤ sight

Note: these number combinations can appear in any position within the SAF chain. For example, a problem with hearing can be indicated in any chain that includes a 5 and a 15.

15-21

If the posterior pituitary (21) is associated with the hypothalamus (15) in a chain, then it is an indicator for an alert study of the pineal body, which secretes melatonin, a hormone that influences sexual maturation and sexual activity.

Emotion: Attention

The emotional correlation to the hypothalamus and the senses can be expressed by the term "attention." It indicates that the person has had repeated distortions of perception or inability to hold concentration for long periods. This trouble comes from both simple and complicated forms of radiation.

We find that when 15 appears in an SAF chain it is a definite sign of degenerative conditions created by excesses of radiation, used in this sense as any particle of energy that moves <u>inward toward the individual</u>.

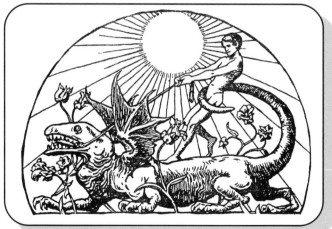

These conglomerated, spliced, conjugated or ephemeral energies can be generated from any source in the environment including other people, other places and even inanimate objects. The emotions are included in this study. For example, if the individual is in a confused situation wherein he has to confront a good deal of

Organs and glands can be considered the friendly dragons of the body as they do immediate work for the complete human system.

> *SAF defines radiational energy as any particle of energy, including emotional, that moves inward toward the individual.*

poignant anger from another party, then the victim or target of this attack is effectively receiving doses of emotional radiation.

Any animate or inanimate object, or any visible or invisible energy approaching inwardly toward a person, is part of sun cycle energy and would be considered radiation. As mentioned previously, any electrical phenomenon now on the planet originated with the sun; therefore, any phenomenon of light (visible or invisible) that seeks the center of an individual can be considered a radiation phenomenon. Each dose of sun cycle energy, in whatever form, must also be considered part of the tally toward a person's aging process.

Scientists and researchers have always been concerned with ionizing radiation, which is of the type that can oxidize tissue, but any form of radiation that increases the stress and pressure to the target system can be counted and must be defended against. When the target system has to kick back against any pressure, the radiation has the ability to confuse and misdirect the overall plan of the body.

Condition: Evaluation

Perhaps the single most important consideration when observing an individual's behavior is his ability to evaluate circumstances. Can he put the proper events in perspective?

Analyzing with the mind (14) is a different factor altogether. Analysis involves dissecting the congealed particles of his pressing problems, whereas in evaluation the individual is putting problems in an order of importance. This order of importance – evaluation – is directly akin to the mathematical actions of the precisely ordered numerical chain of the SAF program.

Many SAF Monitors have noticed tremendous boosts of energy while deciphering and reading numerical chains for other curious individuals. This startling reaction occurs because the forthright practice of studiously evaluating black body masses and black body light explodes the black body light into white body light. This peculiar phenomenon causes unknowns to transform into knowns; mysteries into solved riddles. The effects for both people involved are astounding! An SAF monitor will actually gain energy the more he evaluates and dissects important issues for another person.

So, the numbers 14 and 15 are very important in the consideration of general sanity. It is extremely vital to understand when initiating the practice of SAF that this program moves us directly <u>towards</u> sanity and <u>away from</u> insanity. SAF is the antidote for insanity. The insane individual has become more mentally and physically conglomerated and darkened.

The more black body light we possess the more moronic, stupid and confused we will be. The more white body light we own, the more enlightened and intelligent we will be.

This is why it is mandatory to avoid hypnotic spells, trances or devices that delete our conscious willpower.

We must constantly seek to enhance the capabilities of the individual to judiciously perceive the black body light around him. Hypnotic spells and trances place a darker state of black body light into the person to achieve the goal of the wanton suggestion. Forcing the operator's suggestions into a person's black body light renders that person "suggestible" or "sleepy." The operator of hypnosis will tell the person to make certain he is relaxed and soon he will feel sleepy. Sure enough, the participant feels he is becoming sleepy. And more <u>unconscious</u>.

This is a very dangerous state as far as SAF is concerned. The SAFent working with SAF wants to be more awake, not more asleep. The idea is more self awareness, not less. The darker this black body light becomes, the more the SAFent's energy is turned away from white body light and the easier it is for inhospitable dragons to hide and wait in ambush.

> *Black body light is where all the hungry dragons are patiently hiding.*

Mental Aspects

The hypothalamus (15) is truly a phenomenon born directly out of the spiritual and interpersonal relationships with higher energies and the Supreme Power. To become more godlike, a person must certainly become more aware; he must have as much black body light removed from his system as he can. What is the simplest explanation for <u>white</u> body light? The Supreme Being possesses and controls more white body light than any other being. White body light is intense and powerful. A being of God's magnitude would certainly not have any unconscious areas of his mind, and very few areas of black body mass, if any at all, to understand and perceive all His self-created, mental machinery. Evidently, Earth is one of His mental machines. So, it is a Universal Directive from above and part of humankind's quest to emulate God that makes it imperative that we put our attention on gaining as much white body light as possible.

10-15

If the thyroid (10) and the hypothalamus (15) are together it is an indicator of the black body mass encroaching on the white body light of the individual. If the endocrine system (17/18) is in the same chain, it indicates that dragons are on the move and with them much darkness and confusion will arrive.

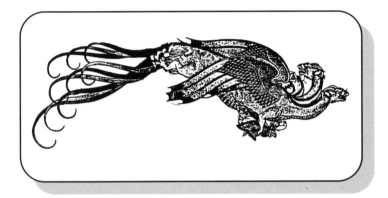

If 10,15 and 17/18 are in the same chain, the dragons are on the move, bringing with them darkness and confusion.

In many cases individuals who possess the 10-15 control numbers have been experiencing a difficult time perceiving through the black body mass. It is difficult to peer through darkness and see accurately.

5-15

When the anterior pituitary (5) is connected with the hypothalamus (15), the individual has a creative sense of distortion. His imagination can go wild inside and around him, causing mental and physical miasma. It becomes difficult to perceive the ideas and mental images that are being transmitted to him from others.

If, for example, someone is talking about a boat with many sails, the distorted person may get an image of a car with leather interior. The garbled and deformed image may be that wild and uncontrollable. Usually this individual, victimized by his own mind, will say, "Huh?" or "What?!!" as if the speaker were crazy! These deformed pictures flash in about 1/20th of a second, they are unbelievably fast, so the person says, "Huh?!" Furthermore, when asking people who have difficulties tracking information around them, we find that many of the plagued individuals' mental memory banks are corroded with dragon-like trauma figures. The particular mental dragons lie sideways across the person's energy pathways and distort his views of his past so that he believes that certain traumatic events had occurred recently when in actuality they didn't happen in this lifetime.

SAF Chains and 5-15 number Combinations

<u>5</u>-<u>15</u>-16-17/18-1-2-4-10-14 ➤ crazy

<u>5</u>-16-17/18-1-2-14-4-<u>15</u> ➤ minor distortion of perception

1-2-4-<u>5</u>-<u>15</u>-20-16-14 ➤ can't distinguish sounds

<u>15</u>-1-2-<u>5</u>-20-16-14 ➤ awakening

2-10-12-<u>15</u>-10-<u>5</u>-13-20 ➤ deep awareness

<u>15</u>-16-22-6-4-20-<u>5</u> ➤ no distortion

10-<u>15</u>-17/18-2-4-6-13-<u>5</u>-1 ➤ learning

1-7-17/18-2-26-4-<u>15</u>-<u>5</u> ➤ truth unveiled in the past

1-2-14-16-20-<u>5</u>-<u>15</u>-17/18-13-10 ➤ can't distinguish words

7-20-24-10-13-16-17/18-8-<u>5</u>-2-<u>15</u> ➤ unsolved mystery

5-10-15-17/18

So the 15-5 sequence in a chain, especially if there is a thyroid (10) and endocrine system (17/18) in the neighborhood (see graph), indicates that there is an intense jumble of dragon life near or in the individual's senses.

When persons with these number combinations are asked about events in the past, they have a very difficult time retrieving them. They have bad recall or no recall at all. Many times someone with these particular numbers (5-15) forgets events that have occurred in the past such as loss of a loved one or certain kinds of traumatic surgical operations, drug taking, etc. He may vehemently deny any of these things ever happened to him! This denial makes matters very confusing for regular practitioners.

SAF Chains with 5-10-15-17/18 Sequences

<u>5</u>-<u>15</u>-<u>10</u>-<u>17/18</u>-22-1-6-24-3 ➤ blocked recall

<u>5</u>-22-<u>15</u>-16-<u>10</u>-20-<u>17/18</u>-2-4 ➤ forgetful

<u>15</u>-<u>5</u>-22-16-<u>10</u>-<u>17/18</u>-20 ➤ amnesia

<u>17/18</u>-20-<u>10</u>-6-9-24-2-<u>15</u>-<u>5</u> ➤ dullard

<u>10</u>-22-<u>15</u>-<u>17/18</u>-6-24-3-5 ➤ dragon bite

1-<u>10</u>-<u>17/18</u>-16-3-<u>5</u>-<u>15</u>-20 ➤ chronic stress

2-<u>5</u>-<u>17/18</u>-<u>10</u>-16-20-<u>15</u>-2-22 ➤ insensitivity to surroundings

1-<u>17/18</u>-20-2-<u>5</u>-<u>10</u>-24-3-<u>15</u> ➤ sympathy sickness

There are many intricate connections of energy involving the number 15 in a numerical chain sequence and it is important to note some of the more delicate ones.

15-17/18

When the endocrine system (17/18) is specifically tied to the hypothalamus (15) then we have what is called "healer's syndrome." These numbers were found to exist in individuals who have inadvertently picked up or absorbed the energy or the twisted ideas of another sick person. Chiropractors and physicians, who work directly with disturbed, diseased or distraught people, contract a good deal of energy by laying their hands on them. The doctors take on some of the actual memories and the conglomerated images of the traumas (dragons) inside the individual's mind and body. It was found that many doctors possessed the same perverted ideas and the bizarre problems of patients they treated. An SAF program called "Physician's Rescue" was developed so that we could actually unravel some of the doctors' traumas and find out which dragons belonged to whom. Doctors often don't realize that many of the problems they are carrying around aren't their own.

15-20

Another signal of mental distortion and the inability to observe reality is when the pancreas (20) falls together with the hypothalamus (15) and creates a 15-20 sequence in an SAF chain. When these numbers are present the individual may be seen to have a very peculiar phenomenon right in the center of the forehead. An invisible knot of energy exists there with such power that it pushes the individual's head backward about 10 degrees. It causes him to look out from under this barrier of energy that is positioned just above his eyes. Many practitioners who have handled or touched people with problems such as cancer, arthritis and heavier diseases have been afflicted with this specific knot in the middle of their foreheads. It appears as a very confused, twisted ball of energy that nestles on the brow. The "doctor's squint," as it is called, comes about because the pressure of this balled black body mass (congealed dragon matter) is enough to squeeze a doctor's capacity to view others into a tiny pinpoint of mass. In order to look through this massive pressure, he has to tilt his head backwards a little.

At the same time, <u>anyone</u> who generates a 15-20 sequence in the chain is liable to have had some pressure buildup in their system, especially in the mind and near the sense mechanisms around the ears, nose, eyes, mouth and even at the tips of the fingers. Epileptics, and those who have observed people in the throes of a seizure or convulsion, will know a manifestation of the 15-20 phenomenon as the "aura." If it were possible to spray this aura with some kind of phosphorescent dye to make it visible to the naked eye, it would resemble a miniature tornado. When this tornado alights on certain parts of the brain or mind, the afflicted individual loses all sense contact with that area.

Physical Aspects

14-15

Regarding physical troubles, we find a similar kind of reaction generated to the rest of the body by the hypothalamus (15) as caused by the mind (14). Tiny tornadoes of energy can light on the body and absolutely foil the present and past energy processes of the body.

11-15

Many times, especially when the veins and arteries (11) are together with the hypothalamus (15), the individual may have hardening of certain body tissues, particularly in the lower half of the body. It is not uncommon for a person to have rectal calculi or kidney stones with 11-15 (see graph). The poisons lodging within the veins and arteries may cause arteriosclerosis and blockages.

SAF Chains and 11-15 combinations often indicate hardening of certain body tissue or stones.

11-15-6-16-22-1-17/18-23 ➤ stones in rectum

6-11-15-16-22-1-23-17/18-3-4 ➤ stones and liver

16-11-15-22-6-5-1-23-4 ➤ stone in kidneys

6-16-1-2-11-15-14-20-22 ➤ chronic stones

1-2-12-5-16-6-14-11-15 ➤ dissolved stones chronic

6-1-2-15-11-7-14-16 ➤ gall bladder stones

11-1-2-16-6-7-14-15 ➤ hemorrhoids and gall bladder dysfunction

---

Solidification of these particular invisible tornadoes of energy is merely the electrical output of dragon entities. Specifically, the trauma that existed in the past is being called up to work on the body in the present, in the <u>now</u>. When a dragon is called up, it breathes fire against the body. These fires come out in the form of tiny tornadoes (Planck's laws of heat, photons, quanta and thermodynamics) that are invisible to the naked eye. But once they infest themselves in the body they stay in there and are able to cause arthritis and calcification in many of the soft tissues.

If an SAF Monitor sees an 11-15 sequence in the chain, he knows that this tornado-like action has been going on a long time and is capable of destroying the tissues within the person's body. If this is the case, we find that many detoxification processes are necessary. Sometimes several dragons will work together on an area of body or mind at the same time just to ensure that the physical parts or mental zone is frozen into place and helpless. The dragons effectively attempt to turn that region of the body or mind into a nest so that they can rapidly reproduce themselves. If the solidification of physical or mental energy is complete enough, they may have gained the ability to procreate.

In essence, what we experience with disease conditions that worsen is the birth of younger dragons. So powerful and so insidious is this process that it infests the genetic system of the human being. These spawned dragons are handed down from one hapless generation of humans to the next.

It seems that the process of existing as a human being is a challenge to unravel this mass of dragon life that has been created by traumatic experiences existing deep in the past of an individual. In other words, we are born with problems that were created by the dragons of past centuries. Some of these are quite formidable.

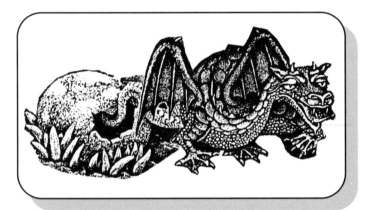

What we experience in disease conditions that worsen is the birth of younger dragons.

To truly reach the state of a super human being, the Übermensch of Carl Jung, we must be able to confront these masterful, powerful and meaningful dragons that have been created by our ancestors.

There are many other influences against number 15 in the stealthy view of a person's case. The number sequences are all-important in detecting this menagerie of "dragondom."

15-16

When the kidneys (16) are together with the hypothalamus (15) in an SAF chain, the individual may have an extraordinary fear of dragons. These two numbers appearing anywhere in the same chain may show that the individual is in retreat from the onslaught of these toxins and poisons. He may be cowardly, afraid of the dragons in his life. Due to the presence of number 16 in the chain, the Monitor should be careful to ascertain whether the SAFent has developed an inability to confront dragons or traumas in his existence. This would be deadly, for the more a person doesn't look at his traumas, the more he has lost his ability to create white body light (the only light that can dissolve dragons). In SAF we welcome trauma dragons because it gives us something to work on. Traumas and the physical representations of trauma, which are the poisons and toxins in a person's body, have power only when they exist in black body light. Therefore, the situation where an individual refuses to look at his problems is a fertile ground for the nesting of dragons in a person's existence.

15-19

When the skin (19) appears with the hypothalamus (15) in the SAF chain, there is a great possibility that the person may be developing a tumor in his body or mind.

The forefathers of medicine, in their attempts to understand when a dragon was impinging upon an individual's body, observed and wrote that particular sequences occurred. Their studies of the physical humors showed that once the toxins invaded the body system and reached the defense mecha-

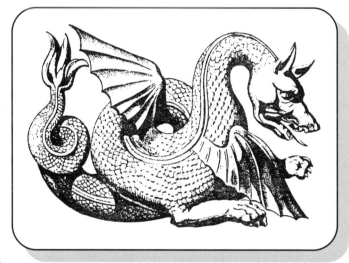

When the hypothalamus connects with the kidneys (15-16), the individual may have an extraordinary fear of the dragons.

nism of the thymus (1), they were effectively <u>in</u>. The ancient scientists called this first step <u>dolar</u> (pain); the second step was <u>rubar</u> (redness), followed by <u>calor</u> (heat), and then after this segment of change an individual would develop a <u>tumor</u> (swelling). Ancient practitioners saw this reaction more or less as a <u>footprint</u> or <u>imprint</u> of an invisible force (black body light) against the body. They understood that they could not <u>see</u> what was making the pain or what was actually making these conditions occur, especially if there was no physical object present, such as a stone or a knife. If a person of that time period suddenly developed a pain or sensation or any kind of mental or physical disorder invisible to the naked eye, then the doctors or practitioners considered that there was some demon or invisible entity involved.

Black body light persists in the presence of white body light because of the ignorance of its existence. It is important to note that these SAF processes are specifically tuned to turn the lights on in the presence of these dragons and take a good look at them. In later chapters of this textbook the author will describe for the reader what a dragon actually looks like. Dragons will be dissected and their intrinsic parts exposed.

15-22

Another number that is important to the physical aspects of the hypothalamus (15) is the parathyroid (22), which shows hardening. The process of creating tumors begins with 15-20, light mass; then 15-21, a tumor that is spongy and made mostly of water; and finally 15-22, a calcified, hardened tumor.

We should have a great deal of respect when viewing a chain with a 15. Radiation and toxins of a black body nature are involved here and we must be very alert to this signal that the SAFent is entering an area that was once dark to him.

SAF Number Combinations with the hypothalamus (15)

5-15 ➤ imagination runs wild

5-15-10-17/18 ➤ poor or no recall (intense jumble of dragons)

10-15 ➤ encroaching black body mass; perception troubles

10-15-17/18 ➤ confusion (dragons are on the move)

11-15 ➤ hardening of body tissues; rectal calculi, kidney stones

15-16 ➤ fear of trauma (dragons)

15-17/18 ➤ healer's syndrome (taking on others dragons)

15-19 ➤ tumors forming

15-20 ➤ light mass tumor; "doctor's squint"; epilepsy; convulsions

15-21 ➤ spongy tumor

15-22 ➤ calcified tumor

16

idneys and
ladder

AT A GLANCE:
Emotion: Fear
Condition: Filtration

The kidneys are a pair of essential organs designated number 16 in SAF. Proper functioning of the kidneys are vital for they filter the blood, remove toxins and excrete the end-product of body metabolism that may otherwise overtax other glands and organs. This end product, urine, is sent to the bladder for storage until voided. The kidneys are resilient. They regulate the concentrations of minerals and other ions in the extracellular fluid.

Emotion: Fear

When the number 16 appears in a specific chain sequence, the SAFent correspondingly exhibits an acute or chronic fear or phobia. However, the position of the number 16 in the chain determines phobic action. There may be circumstances involving acute terror of specific dangers. Whenever 16 appears in a chain, it indicates that the dragons of a person's life situations have caused a constant fear for the confrontation of the dragons themselves.

Sometimes those who exhibit the number 16 in a numerical chain have a difficult time realizing that they even have traumas. Not being able to express or confront these dragons causes a great deal of pain and sensation. However, the fear of trauma (dragon) can't be classified as a trauma itself. In various circumstances persons who have fear

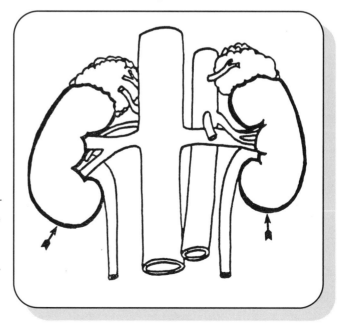

Kidneys

reactions will exhibit the number 16 in an SAF chain. Fear reactions are a specific organizing of human energy that tries desperately to escape an environmental or mental/physical danger.

The problem arises when the person has traumatic dragons buried in the deep subconscious that cause the individual his true fears. In other words, phobias are stacked one on top of another like a deck of 3-D playing cards. If you have a particular phobia, such as fear of animals or insects, you will have other phobias underneath these fears that you can't see. This has been the understanding, the breakthrough and the rule made by SAF. SAF technicians have been able to uncover the real poisonous or toxic situation underneath the outer crust of trauma, which gives rise to other false or misdiagnosed conditions.

Condition: Filtration

The actions of the kidneys are part of a purposeful chromosomal objective. Any entity or structure of living organism in the environment must have the ability to filter out toxins; however, these may sometimes be mislabeled. And because a person can't discern a toxin from a friendly bit of energy, he may sometimes become confused and erroneously allow a villain into his system. The kidneys are very specific in their action. They act like a deft screen. They take poisons out of a polluted blood stream and remove the byproducts of metabolism to thoroughly cleanse the human machine.

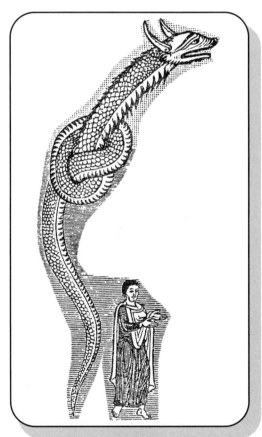

The kidneys act much as an oil filter does in a car. Dirt is considered the primary enemy of any machine, computer or body-mechanism. If poisons, dust and dirt get into a body, the resultant motion of these materials within the dirty blood can easily cause an abrasion of the internal structure of organs, glands, cells and tissues, thereby wearing down the system. Once toxins, dirt and poisons get into the organs, the organs are easy targets for destruction. This is because noxious substances can swiftly infiltrate delicate

Many times individuals who exhibit number 16 in a chain have a difficult time realizing they have traumas.

places in the body and embed themselves so it is important that the kidneys endlessly create this filtration mechanism.

16-22

When the kidneys (16) are found in an SAF chain with the parathyroid (22) there is a definite possibility that non-specific toxins and poisons within the system are beginning to solidify and take up root. As relayed previously, the dragons or traumatic situations of past scenarios can certainly create a miniature tornado-like effect in the invisible realms, between visible physical dimensions, and can ultimately build up masses. These radiant but condensed masses are powerful enough to create concretions affixed to the walls of soft tissue. This may seem to be a more unusual circumstance or an exception, but it is quite common in humanoids.

The combination of kidneys (16) and parathyroid (22) show poisons are beginning to take root

1-2-5-<u>16</u>-<u>22</u>-10-15-19-24 ➤ Kidney Stones

<u>16</u>-3-4-7-10-20-13-23-17/18-<u>22</u> ➤ Kidney Discomfort

<u>22</u>-1-3-5-23-24-15-20-<u>16</u> ➤ No Stones

4-10-<u>16</u>-17/18-20-<u>22</u>-1-2-5-8 ➤ Kidneys Weak

9-<u>22</u>-23-<u>16</u>-12-13-20-14-15-24-1 ➤ Gravel

2-<u>16</u>-8-4-5-10-<u>22</u> ➤ Stones Hardening

6-24-17/18-4-20-13-<u>16</u>-<u>22</u> ➤ Stones in the Past

5-2-7-6-8-<u>22</u>-<u>16</u>-24-1-10-13 ➤ Dissolved Stones

The layering or depositing of energy in one location will definitely cause the existence or the creation of mass. It is the audacity of the chemically-biased dragon to reproduce itself so much in one location that it actually comes out of the black body light in which it usually exists and becomes <u>visible</u> in white body light. In this case, the dragon sneers at the thymus (1). He sometimes will laugh because he has won for the moment; he has occupied a space in the visible light spectrum. These dragons are called tumors, stones and other names and they will show up from time to time.

It is essential for any individual practicing SAF to understand that the visualization or realization of energy in a solid state is merely the compilation of minute radiant energies that have piled themselves onto one location and one spot at one time. These tiny phenomena of stones, parasites, toxins, vermin and other pests that invade the body are merely the end result of many hours, days, months and years, even centuries of accumulations of energies in one place at one time.

The creation mechanism of a kidney stone, for example, is the same kind of mechanism used to create a human being, an animal, a bird, an insect or any other life form on the planet. The key is the eternal application of energies to one spot. The energies must collide into one location and create a swirling pattern like an invisible, diminutive tornado that ultimately wraps around itself like a ball of string and becomes visible.

This action occurs in the reproduction of human beings. When the sperm invades the egg and a zygote is formed, the energy begins to wrap around itself and create a tornado-like effect. The fetus, in the early stages of pregnancy, appears coiled into itself, wrapped up. As the fetus grows, these tornadoes of invisible energy become powerful enough in that location that they can finally unravel themselves.

It is the same principle when dragons form in the shape of stones and tumors. The entity that invades the body is strong enough to create a tornado of energy, which wraps around itself. Ultimately, if a kidney stone or any other kind of anomaly were allowed to persist, it would mold into the visage of the dragon itself. In other words, those particular entities are the offspring of the dragon, the true marriage or collision of life forms that fostered it. Particles that grow into stones are "dragon eggs" being laid in a person's body. If they are given enough time they can become the exact duplicate of the dragon, a 3-Dimensional hologram of a trauma that may have existed ancestrally eons ago.

What many people don't understand about dragons is that traumatic situations don't usually take on the gruesome appearance of a snarling, fire-breathing lizard with a pointed tail and leathery wings. The dragons that live in this text are those created by the collision of various energies in the environment against the human being.

Often dragons take on the appearance of car bumpers that have crushed the individual in the past, or the appearance of stairs, baseball bats, familiar faces of women or men, the vision of a childhood house. All manner of animate and inanimate objects that have collided with the human being are encased in a protective photographic state so that they can prolong and proliferate their existence.

On the other hand, many dragons are the visage of humanoids or of monsters and demons. SAFents have been confronted by all manner of living forms on the planet. Whatever a person visualizes as his dragon, has certainly become his dragon.

People fear insects, even tiny little bugs, because throughout the centuries the genetic blueprint of the body has recorded attacks by insects. When a body is put into the ground the cells are still alive. As the bugs and crawly creatures come to devour the

> *Whatever a person visualizes as his dragon, has certainly become his dragon.*

last vestiges of that human being, those genetic cells are still recording the trauma of being eaten alive by a very large creature, such as a worm or a beetle. To the genetic program, in a state of being devoured underground, a bug will appear to be 30 or 40 feet tall in comparison to the cell. Hence, many people have a dread of creepy crawly bugs, roaches, worms, spiders and the like.

This type of phenomenon is part of the kidney reaction; the kidney itself developed a fear of being unable to reject a toxin. Many of the poisons that are filtered from the kidneys are sent immediately to the bladder. Compared to the colon (3), which has more strength, the kidneys are daintier and more frightened when it comes to disposing of byproducts.

When severely frightened, a basic human reaction is the tendency to urinate. The phrase "that scared the piss out of him" is descriptive of this. When a person becomes fearful, the fluid carrying many of the unwanted materials are rejected very rapidly. The reason for this: no two fears can occupy the same space at the same time. The body actually trades one fear for another. The toxins that are in the body in the form of urine, urea, etc. are less detrimental to the system than an unknown perhaps greater fear, so the body trades off the lesser fear, the urine, by releasing it. Of course to create this circumstance someone has to be terrorized into letting go.

16-20

When the kidneys (16) are associated with the pancreas (20), this may be a signal that the kidneys' center of gravity is off balance and poisons are escaping into the body system. There may be a dragon infesting the kidneys of the type that creates inflammation. In many cases this has been staidly reviewed by medical science as Bright's Disease. The affected person passes albumen via his urine and complains of a definite dysfunction of normal kidney processes.

SAF Chains and 16-20 Combinations

1-3-5-7-<u>16</u>-<u>20</u>-8-9-10-24 ➤ Kidney Infection

<u>16</u>-1-3-5-7-8-9-10-<u>20</u> ➤ Kidney Dysfunction

<u>20</u>-10-1-3-5-9-7-8-24-<u>16</u> ➤ No Kidney Dysfunction

<u>16</u>-<u>20</u>-3-6-9-7-1-2-4-6-24 ➤ Kidney Pain

14-<u>16</u>-17/18-10-<u>20</u>-13-12-4-19-21 ➤ Chronic Kidney Trouble

2-4-6-8-9-<u>20</u>-13-15-<u>16</u>-7 ➤ Intermittent Kidney Trouble

15-16

When the kidneys (16) join with the hypothalamus (15) in an SAF chain, a greenish tint to the urine may indicate hemoglobin is being lost through urination. Hemoglobin is the material that carries the iron, laden with oxygen, through the body. The 15-16 sequence is an indicator that the person may be becoming magnetically polarized, as the dipole revolves near the trauma site in the body. Some energy in the environment powerful enough to electrically sway iron in the body may have come into the vicinity. A dragon forceful enough to cause the blood to change course must be recognized and handled. Often when a 15-16 is in the chain it indicates that the person may be under the control of barbaric dragon influences. This state can be verified if the person behaves in a zombie-like fashion.

16-any organ number

When the number 16 is present in an SAF chain, the SAFent and Monitor should look to the target organ. Proper filtration of noxious substances in each organ is mandatory for tissue and cell survival. If an organ or gland complex allows toxins and poisons to escape into its tissues, then it will reduce the efficiency or output of that particular organ complex.

SAF number combinations with kidneys (16):

15-16 ➤ Hemoglobin in urine (person becoming magnetically polarized)

16-20 ➤ Bright's Disease – Albumin in urine (kidneys' center of gravity is off balance and poisons escape into system)

16-21 ➤ Kidney Stones (Poisons in system begin to solidify)

Mental Aspects

Probably the most pernicious mental aspect of the presence of 16 in a chain is the reality of fears, phobias and terrors. A 16 shows the person has a definite unwillingness to confront certain circumstances in the environment. A person's face sometimes can reveal the degree of fear present. The tone of the skin, bags under the eyes, pallor, cachexia, lines, wrinkles and a haggard look are indicators. Swollen eyes are often a clue. It tags a person who may have a specific fear or problem confronting certain subjects.

There is a plethora of listed phobias in medical science that involves every kind of action imaginable. A phobia indicates the person is unable to handle a particular mass, energy, or concept (any or all of these). The rest of this text will depict the actions of environmental reminders that may trigger all manner of phobic reactions.

It was determined with SAF programming that what the person actually fears is not the real problem. The mechanism of the "reminder" contends that the SAFent is looking at a white body mass, some visible energy, which is serving as a trigger or reminder for some black body mass or black body creature (a dragon). This dragon or trauma, beneath the SAFent's awareness, is using light body energy or creatures in the present environment to trigger thoughts of itself (the trauma or dragon). The way that it does this is very simple.

A specific energy in the environment (such as the color of a person's hair) can be similar to that of the beast (who may have the same hair color) that lies within the person's unconscious. This mechanism is able to stimulate a person's memory enough to awaken the dragon from his sleep and cause him (the dragon) to go into action. Now when dragons (traumas) are put into action, they infest, pervade and invade the nervous system, producing symptomatology. They create pains, sensation and discomfort, and they cause headaches, nausea, vomiting, nervousness and all of the basic problems of man.

You might ask why a dragon would want to be awakened from his rest. Wouldn't he much rather have a nice quiet sleep? Dragons are able to go through existence undisturbed, but in reality the extent of their existence depends upon the amount of playing time they receive. In other words, each time a stimulated dragon plays out his dark existence or sends his arcane message to his human host, he etches the groove of a macabre recording into that unwary human being a little bit deeper. So the number of times the dragon's scenario is played gives it maturity or tenure in the body.

The playing of the excited dragon is vital to the existence or perpetuity of the phobia because dragons must be played or they may be forgotten altogether. They must be played out of black body light, for if they appear in white body light form, they will summarily be destroyed. (This can be demonstrated in the lore of Dracula, who was never allowed to come into the light or he would be vaporized. The dragon has a similar script.)

The fact is that if a dragon is to get a "play," he must nudge or work his host into a space where the host can have a "reminder." A reminder is extremely important because if the dragon doesn't have a reminder then he doesn't get a "play" and if he doesn't get a "play," then he won't be fed. In other words, to feed a dragon, we must find a reminder for him.

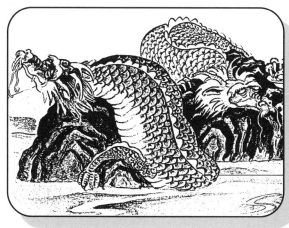

Dragons must be played or they may be forgotten altogether. They must be played out of their black body light homes into white body light so they can be summarily destroyed (vaporized).

The dragons can only get their nourishment from the present time because that is where all the actual live energy is located. The present time contains all the light energy and knowing energy. A dragon can't know or express his own existence unless he is fed by the present time, so it is vital for him to involve individuals in situations similar to the dragon himself so that these reminders can feed him.

Consider a person who is accident-prone. They have been able, by some "coincidence," to injure the same body part over and over again. Such actions are merely the dragon getting the person into situations where he will be reminded of the same trauma. The dragon gets play and thus gets energy.

For example, you may have hurt your foot when you were younger. Suppose you were playing baseball and someone wearing a cleat stepped on your foot. In this particular case, your "dragon" may look like a shoe with points. We could say that a baseball shoe with cleats makes a fine dragon. The cleats could be the teeth and the stitching could be the eyes, and from up close, it would be a very formidable looking dragon! You will see reminders all around so the dragon can have a "play." You will subsequently get into similar, unhappy situations. Perhaps you (the SAFent) could drop a book on the same foot or trip and fall on the same foot, or you could stub your toe on the side of your bed. These recurrent collisions give the dragon more energy, more power. If you have the particular trouble of having a dragon like that, you must look for anything that reminds you of the dragon/trauma in the first place. If it were a shoe with cleats, you would have to find something that looked like a shoe. In this scenario it is difficult to get away from reminders because we have to wear shoes every day. Each time a shoe is put on, it would be one reminder or one "play" for the dragon. You would find yourself in a chronic situation where you would be endlessly replaying the dragon's scene and be in the unique jeopardy of having accidents occur to that same body part.

Fear now kicks in because you are unable to control this dragon miasma; you live in a constant state of phobic symptomatology wherein you feel chills and scary sensations such as dizziness and vertigo. You feel the kickback of your own genetic diagram telling you to get out of the way because the dragon is coming. The genetic program itself works in black body light, so it can help avert dragon feeding problems and cause you, the dauntless but stupefied individual, to get out of the way.

We experience much symptomatology in the presence of a hungry dragon, for the dragon (trauma) is actually trying to encroach on the space of the genetic blueprint. The genetic cells, the DNA/RNA and the chromosomes feel the invasion of this wily trauma (dragon) as it tries to install its own existence and purpose. A dragon with the image of a shoe with cleats might try to cause the related body part (the foot) to spawn dragons of the same nature. We can imagine what they would look like if they were able to develop into that particular dragon-visage. Many people develop foot problems slowly; first they experience extreme tenderness, then sores, and later bunions will form within casts of calcium that bend and twist. Under a high powered microscope, they look more and more like a spike or a cleat. When that dragon has enough "plays" it has the power to create or reproduce, to have "children."

6-16

If the kidneys (16) are joined by the liver (6) in an SAF chain, then the SAFent may be experiencing the fear of change. In such a case, you have grown so accustomed to them, you may be afraid to change your problems. It is a fear primarily coming from dragon talk. The dragons, of course, certainly don't want you to fix your problems or your case conditions because many of them come directly from the dragons themselves. When such "dragon talk" goes on in your mind, you may prevent yourself from doing SAF chains or <u>any</u> programs for your betterment. You will likely speak your fears and phobias because you don't want to change. You may be afraid that if you lose your dragons, your problems, you will lose your life, your existence, or your personality. We have to compromise somewhat with someone who has these problems because he or she is not "all together" in his head. The dragons are more or less thwarting this person.

This same number combination (6-16) indicates that the person will have trouble in any situation where change is taking place, such as in divorce, separation, losses, business troubles, etc. The person will have a difficult time coping. This change of energy or change of location is detrimental to the person's existence because it acts as a reminder and causes a "play" for his dragon, giving the dragon much more power. In other words, the dragon is saying in this case, "See, I told you this would happen to you and that you would lose."

Often the dragon was originally created in a traumatic circumstance, one in which the individual was connected to a heavy, horrible loss experience in the past. It may have started with his parents, then through time, places and events were recorded where he himself had failed. This new change (loss of the dragon) may constantly remind him that he is losing and he is going to be taken advantage of again.

13-16

If the kidneys (16) combine with the adrenal glands (13), the SAFent may have a problem or a phobia dealing with the performance of spectacular or heroic actions. He may even have a fear of being unable to accomplish very ordinary deeds. In many cases, 13-16 in a numerical chain indicates that the person may have trouble facing projects he has put together because he is afraid they won't succeed. He is the type who says, "Well, I'm not sure that this is going to work out for me, and if I invest my money and time I'm going to lose. I'll fail anyway." A person with this particular SAF chain combination may already be aware of his phobias about future plans and projects.

Failure is always a dragon.

SAF chains and 13-16 combinations

1-2-4-6-10-23-15-14-<u>13-16</u> ➤ Failed Long Ago

<u>13-16</u>-24-17/18-6-7-8-1-5 ➤ Recent Failure

2-4-10-20-13-16-5-3-7-9 ➤ Failed Plan

<u>13</u>-1-2-3-4-5-6-0-21-17/18-<u>16</u> ➤ Possible Failure

<u>16</u>-22-10-14-12-1-2-20-<u>13</u> ➤ Success (numbers are reversed.)

2-4-6-8-<u>13</u>-20-5-7-9-<u>16</u> ➤ Chronic Failure

3-6-<u>16</u>-20-21-22-24-<u>13</u>-17/18 ➤ Intermittent Failure

2-1-10-12-<u>13</u>-14-<u>16</u>-20-22-23 ➤ Worried about Failure

A 13-16 type is stuck in a rut and is a prisoner of his own program. If the 13-16 appears to the extreme right of the SAF chain, he has had failure in the past. His mind is still stuck on this and the failure scene is his dragon. Failure is always a dragon, and this dragon may have many heads, each head holding the image of a person involved in his failure. This chimera is attached to a hydrous body that is so energetically charged that anytime the host tries a new or fresh project, this multi-headed beast attacks him and flunks him like a school marm who sat on a chair full of tacks. Furthermore, if he tries to get away from this dragon, the dragon convinces him he will be destroyed in the goriest way imaginable. A horrendously sad feeling then envelops the host because all he can do is feed the dragon.

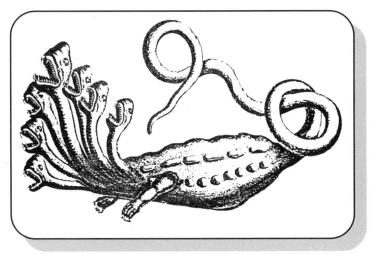

The failure dragon may have many heads, each head holding the image of a person involved in the individual's failure.

Every time he makes a plan, every time he has a desire or a dream and tries to make it come true, he unwittingly calls up this ugly beast to feed on him. It is very disconcerting to have something so formidable in the path of our energies. It causes us to stay away from the idea that we will ever amount to anything. Therefore, we stop ourselves from succumbing and push ourselves into a grind like some mindless laborer in Hades. We plant ourselves into what we believe to be a safe routine, one that is dragon-sanctioned. We become dull, robotic, and uninterested in anything. We are now "the victim," and we complain to others that our life is useless and boring. As we complain we harbor and feed this extremely fascinating and interesting dragon that waits in a black body closet. If we would ever let this dragon out or actually showed it to anyone, we would be the most sought after person in the world; but of course, the dragon will never come out in the daylight to show itself. It always exists in the shadows and stays away.

Physical Aspects

When an individual gets sharp back pains or notices troubles with his eyes (e.g. bags under the eyes) or fluids building up in different areas of the body, the kidneys are to blame. The posterior pituitary (21) also helps establish the body's correct water balance. Because water is the perfect conductor, it is the human system's molecular construction that can cause discomfort. It is important to make sure that the surface tension of the water in the body, plus the purity of the water, is maintained.

> ### Detoxification:
>
> lungs (7)   = gas detoxification
> kidneys (16) = water detoxification
> colon (3)   = solid detoxification

Many times when an individual complains of skin trouble (19), he is probably experiencing some deep trouble with the kidneys (16), the lungs (7), or the colon (3). The important notion to remember is that the lungs (7) take care of all gas detoxification; the kidneys (16) take care of all the body's water detoxification; and the colon (3) takes care of all the body's solids. If all three organs are working properly then the levels of gas, liquid and solid in the body are being properly detoxified.

The final area from where all toxins eventually exit, is the skin (19), the body's outer encasement. As we exhale (7) the breath must go beyond the skin; as we urinate (16) the urine must go beyond the skin; as we defecate (3) the feces must go outside the skin.

1-16

When the thymus (1) associates with the kidneys (16), then some energy or poison has worked its way into the system. Of course, the thymus (1) is indicative of the highest pressure possible, so that if an infection or inflammation is invading the kidneys, it means that the toxin or the trauma is powerful enough to take up root there and actually disrupt the detoxification process.

In all physical aspects involving the kidneys, we should make sure that the kidneys themselves are clear. Just as we are careful to change the oil, gas and air filters in a car, so we should be mindful that the filter of the body – the kidneys – are properly detoxifying.

4-16

If a person is casting off urine filled with proteinaceous substances, he must worry that there is some kind of breakdown in the filtering process. This is because the digestion (4) is erratic. When we see a (4) in a numerical chain along with a (16), we should realize that there is some kind of toxic situation being created because the digestion is off.

1-16-20

If the pancreas (20) connects with the kidneys (16) and the thymus (1) in an SAF chain, there may be a definite problem involving the indigestibility of toxins and poisons, not to mention foods, solids, liquids and gases.

SAF Chains and 4-16 combinations

4-16-20-15-2-10-17/18-24 ➤ Indigestible Matter
20-15-2-10-17/18-24-23-4-16 ➤ Never Digested
4-20-15-2-10-17/18-24-16 ➤ Possible Indigestion
16-20-15-2-10-17/18-24-23-4 ➤ No Indigestion
1-23-22-24-4-16-2-10-17/18-15 ➤ Fear Of Indigestion
2-10-3-5-16-4-20-23-17/18-24 ➤ Phobia
1-2-3-4-13-20-16-17/18-19-23 ➤ Chronic Indigestion
1-5-16-20-13-22-23-4-6-8 ➤ Intermittent Indigestion

SAF Chains with 1-16-20 combinations

1-16-20-4-5-15-23-24-22 ➤ Toxic Wastes
2-4-3-6-10-15-5-23-1-16-20 ➤ Chronic Toxic Waste
1-2-3-6-5-16-17/18-15-22-4-20 ➤ Possible Toxins
7-8-3-6-1-16-20-15-22-4-10 ➤ Toxic Syndrome
20-22-3-4-16-17/18-14-15-20-1 ➤ No Toxins
1-16-5-6-7-9-10-20 ➤ Kidney Poisons
16-20-10-22-15-16-17/18-2-3-1 ➤ Kidney Infection
16-22-23-20-5-6-1 ➤ Chronic Kidney Trouble
10-1-20-15-22-23-17/18-16 ➤ Chronic Poison

17/18

ndocrine System

The endocrine system consists of the glands and organs considered the <u>power train</u> – the anterior pituitary and the hypothalamus (the master organs and glands of the body), the thyroid, the adrenal glands, the pancreas and the sex organs.

This system is considered part of that sequence of energy that causes us to look and behave the way we do. It is the mechanism that creates structure and processes energy. This framework of glands helps all other glands and organs in their daily functions. In a sense, the remaining organs, the liver, heart, spleen, etc., are merely servomechanisms for this power train.

Both numbers 17 and 18 are used for this organ complex; number 17 represents male hormones while number 18 represents female hormones. This sequence, 17/18, is extremely important because of its ability to track dragons. When the 17/18 shows itself in the numerical chain, it is indicative that a trauma or a dragon is stimulated and has occurred in a precise region of a person's past. A numerical chain, because it is a layered and stratified past history, will give the present time on the left side of the chain and the past on the right. So wherever the 17/18 falls in the SAF chain sequence, it will give us a better idea of exactly where the significant traumas have been created in time.

Emotion: Conservative

The endocrine system (17/18) must be balanced so we can produce power.

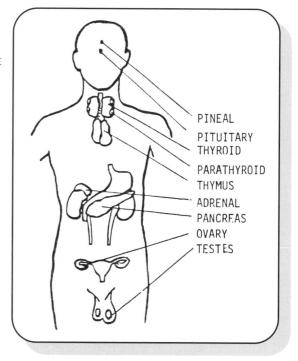

PINEAL
PITUITARY
THYROID
PARATHYROID
THYMUS
ADRENAL
PANCREAS
OVARY
TESTES

The Endocrine System

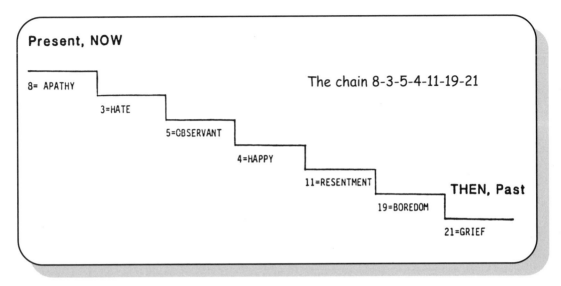

Present, NOW

The chain 8-3-5-4-11-19-21

8= APATHY

3=HATE

5=OBSERVANT

4=HAPPY

11=RESENTMENT

THEN, Past

19=BOREDOM

21=GRIEF

A numerical chain, because it is a layered and stratified past history of the person, will give the present time on the left side of the chain and the past on the right.

Without an organized and aligned endocrine system, there may not be sufficient usable power. Energy failures occur because we have had a trauma in the past. In other words, the dragons are able to cause us to lean toward one set of hormones or the other.

Ferocious dragons that have the right stuff to create disruptive pressure, such as those demons that are created out of automobile accidents and drug abuse, encrust into the fertile body. Pressure-packed dragons control the male hormones; dragons born out of degradations, embarrassment and loss will impress themselves on the female organs or female hormones. This sets up a very interesting situation inasmuch as the hormone mechanisms of the body control not only the temperament of the individual, but also all the secondary sex characteristics.

If a person is abused enough by pressure circumstances, male dragons will be created. The male hormones will be compromised and the individual may have more receptive or masochistic feminine qualities. On the other hand, if more losses are present, and the individual finds that he is being hit with more female dragons, then he may turn the other way and have more of an aggressive, sadistic male personality.

Dragons are able to infest the hormone structure, creating a definite effeminate or masculine quality in certain individuals, because of the abuse and trauma that affect the hormone-producing mechanisms. By understanding the production and inhibition of the hormones testosterone (male) and estrogen (female), we can predict the creation of homosexuality in men and lesbianism in females. These states exist primarily because male or female dragons have taken up a certain space in the body.

The SAF science is very simplistic in this respect. Suppose a male dragon has taken up residence and is active in a male body. By following the laws of chemistry and physics, where two objects can't occupy the same space at the same time, one force must be kicked out. So, if the male dragon presence is crowding or inhibiting the male hormone production, then estrogen will reign supreme. On the other hand, if a person has been hit with a female dragon (losses), then testosterone will reign supreme. This can happen in the case of males or females.

Psychologically, if a man has had tremendous pressure brought to bear and had to admit defeat via a crushing effect of some impact from the environment, then he may become weak and effeminate. On the other hand, if in a male body an individual has been struck with female dragons and many losses, then he may develop more masculine qualities. The same principle would apply to females.

This is not to simplify the problems created by hormone imbalances, only to give a basic premise as to the distortion of them. Male and female dragons can hit a person simultaneously and affect one or the other system in tandem. If an individual has these particular hormone imbalances from some traumatic impact of the past, he has been programmed by the male (pressure) or female (loss/space) dragon to perform in a certain characteristic way. The process is complicated and may involve whole families of dragons or a whole species of dragon that enter human beings. It also may come from a dragon that is part of a virus or bacteria that roams the earth. It has been found in SAF programming that if an individual maintains a conservative output and is unable to perform to his fullest capabilities and talents, or if he is reluctant to move into higher states of energy, then he must be harboring some male or female dragon. This particular balance of male versus female, aggressiveness versus receptivity, is extremely important. It guides the manner of treatment. (see also *AIDS: The Final piece to the Puzzle.*)

Condition: Equalize

The 17/18 embodies all the most important functions and ramifications of energy necessary to understand all sciences, not just SAF. The dichotomy of male and female is carried throughout each science. For instance, in chemistry, male and female is depicted by <u>acid</u> (male) and <u>alkaline</u> (female). In physics, <u>radiation</u> is the male idea and <u>gravitation</u> is female. In astrophysics, <u>pressure</u> is considered male and <u>space</u> is female. In Chinese medicine, <u>yang</u> denotes male, and <u>yin</u> is female.

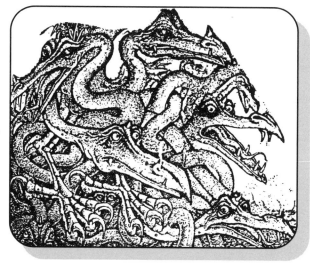

The process of programming an individual may involve whole families of dragons or a whole species.

When 17/18 appears in the chain it automatically indicates this individual has lost his balance or perception for the basic dichotomies of life. "To be or not to be" is the basic question. To exist or not to exist. To perform or not to perform. The basic questions of existence, mobility and intelligence are brought forward when 17/18 is encrusted into a chain.

15–17/18

When 17/18 is connected with the hypothalamus (15) in a numerical chain, it is imperative to understand that the SAFent is sensing, evaluating or studying one of his own traumas. In a sense, when trying to decipher a trauma, we contact reminders in other people. We may very easily cry because someone else is crying. Strangers sobbing on a television program can trigger our trauma. Even when confronted with the fact that the television people we mourn have absolutely nothing in common with our life, it won't change things one iota because this radiant scene feeds a dragon. If we watch someone crying on television or in the same room, we can be instantly reminded of a traumatic situation in which we cried. But the consequences of this action are subtler than an outburst of tears. A person can be picking up reminders from just about any source. This can only happen because our hormones are physically, mentally, and spiritually (mass, energy, concept) out of balance. Many times, however, mere hormone indications on chemical tests are not enough. We may have a perfect report on a blood test and still be unbalanced. Remember that energy is 99% invisible, and the hormone balances on the harmonic levels of radiational energy in the body may be distorted in many different areas. For example, radio waves, sound waves or microwaves on other levels in the body would not show up on a chemical test; and dragons, like poltergeists, are plucky enough to change their settings while the test is being taken. Many patients get a clean bill of health when they go to the medical doctor because medical science is not programmed to scan all aspects of energy. These patients are still uncomfortable and "know" something is wrong even though the mechanic (doctor) didn't "hear the noise" when the patient ran his engine (body) for him.

14-17/18

When 17/18 is found connected with the mind (14) in a chain, there is a very difficult situation to observe. The individual has a common but nasty dragon present. The mind itself is a series of connecting black body masses that are only ignited by white body masses of attention (15) when the individual calls for them. In other words, all the mind's material remains hidden in black body masses until it is ready to be recalled. When data is recalled, the specific overseer of the mind – the spirit – is able to shed light on a certain area and re-illuminate it. People unable to recall certain memories are said to have a bad memory, however, the ability to recall might be blocked by an impudent dragon. Once we are able to illuminate the mind, we can see all our memories – pleasant and unpleasant. These mind files are quite formidable and vast. But first we must control insubordinate dragons that rob us from remembering things. Dragons, again, are created by traumas of collision and loss. These are the poisons in the environment. So, if you were infested with these remembrances, your memory would be very poor. When the mind (14) is connected with the endocrine system (17/18) in a SAF chain, you may have a very difficult time ridding yourself of memory dragons. Your mind may be unable to illuminate the dragons in the proper perspective.

The 14-17/18 sequence indicates that the person is having business troubles. He has business and economy troubles of the mind. He can't order his mind. His mind has altered what is significant. Many times he may put his attention on things that are not important and ponder them, causing himself a gross worry. When we see a 14-17/18 sequence in the chain, we see a person who has had difficulty in maintaining the economy of his life. He is not able to utilize his energy to the fullest extent. He wastes his energy. He finds himself in positions where people can easily take advantage of him.

Look at the 14-17/18 chain combinations. If the 14-17/18 is farther down to the right of the chain it indicates that in the past the SAFent has been abused. He may say, "I have been ripped off." His own dragons have caused him to be ripped off. His own basic traumas have led him into the trap of being disabled so that <u>they</u> could be fed. People believe energy can be bad because they can't discern who or what is trying to hurt them, in this case the dragon. Dragons are only trying to survive; there is a race for space.

SAF Chains and 14-17/18 Combinations

<u>14-17/18</u>-15-23-1-2-10-5-7 ➤ business trouble

1-2-10-15-23-5-<u>14-17/18</u> ➤ failed business

2-10-1-5-<u>14-17/18</u>-23-22-8 ➤ worried about business

1-2-<u>17/18</u>-15-<u>14</u>-23-10-5-7 ➤ chronic business trouble

<u>17/18</u>-2-8-10-21-23-<u>14</u> ➤ no business trouble

<u>14</u>-4-5-6-20-11-9-8-<u>17/18</u> ➤ possible financial ruin

1-<u>17/18</u>-20-2-4-9-15-<u>14</u>-8 ➤ start of financial success

---

It is a very curious phenomenon, but when we finally sort it all out, the dragons really mean us no harm. Dragons need space. We can help the dragons exist in a whole other place and time similar to them – one where they are not interfering or intersecting with our energies. If we can get the dragons away from the body we certainly can help ourselves and help the dragons too. There is no way that we can destroy energy, including dragon energy. It is a non-erasable, non-destroyable substance. The memory of something lives on forever. What we certainly can do, however, is edit our viewpoint of the dragon. We can change our mind about our conditions. We can change the importance and the significance of those things that we believe are in our way.

Many sciences today are trying to help mankind rid themselves of dragons. Many preach that the dragons are "bad" and they have to be eliminated. They must be destroyed because they're a lot of trouble. The dragons, however, can't be erased; they can only be banished. It is the human's energy bank account that the dragon has accessed; this is the power that the dragon uses that the SAFent can take back. The dragon entity is an idea that goes on forever. It has no time and no space.

There is no way that we can get rid of the <u>idea</u> of a dragon. We can, however, get rid of the power the dragon has over the body, mind and spirit, which is a great accomplishment in itself.

When we understand that power and energy created in this environment is all <u>good</u> and for the benefit of everyone, then we become more understanding of this endocrine system (17/18). We must learn how to coordinate all energies, friends and enemies alike, and also be able to control all factors of energy.

In most cases, a person will have enemies in his environment. There may be people, places, and objects that vie for the same space at the same time. They will try to take energy away from him. There might be someone who is trying to take his best girl away, or maybe there is a situation that may take the things he loves away from him. These are problems of space ownership.

People who are enemies on a lower scale could be allies on a grander scale. If a crisis arose where the future of the entire country was at stake, everyone would have to band together to stop the common enemy from invading and taking everyone's freedom and space.

If we are coordinated and understand the energy mechanisms of life to the fullest extent we will realize that all energies will fit into the proper perspective. We don't alter that perspective to make it fit just for us and our own diminutive dimension. We don't become selfish, but do become more determined to see that every energy in the universe is balanced and coordinated and fits the master blueprint. In this way we can never be harmed. We can never be hurt.

There is no dragon big enough to hurt a person who is constantly maintaining the order of the universe, who is constantly striving to see that all cosmos is propagated. Chaos immediately drops away from any situation that is brought into the presence of order and harmony.

13-17/18

If the endocrine system (17/18) is connected with the adrenal glands (13), then the individual has a creation problem. He has lost his zest for living. The encroachment of the dragons has been so severe and his perspective so lost on the energy within his system, that the black body masses infest his very existence to capture the space of his body and mind. This take-over can interfere with the very process of seeing and controlling the dragons. To eliminate dragon power and put dragons in their perspective cages, we must understand their origin. When 13-17/18 are together, it shows that the person has all but given up hope. He has lost the courage to face his dragons.

12-17/18

When the endocrine system (17/18) is connected with the brain (12) then the individual may be exhibiting some pattern of allergy within his system. He is trying to reject toxins and poisons. He is trying to kick out the black body masses invading his nervous system, believing that foods taken into his system are responsible for the feeding of these black body masses or dragons. He may be extremely confused. The actions of eating are being confused with the reminding system of the dragons. This person has developed a dragon complex that may be overwhelming.

10-17/18

When the endocrine system (17/18) is associated with the thyroid (10) the person may have a good deal of intolerable stress. He may be unable to cope with these situations at all. His system may build up fat barriers or insulation around the endocrine system. All his organs may be encrusted with fat deposits because fatty substances are able to thwart dragons from chewing up the organs. Because the dragons use megawatt lightning to disturb the endocrine system, the body will, in defense, put crude fat into all his systems and cause a definite disability of the body to ground itself against this dragon energy. Therefore, the electrical impulses of the dragon can't move through and create havoc in the endocrine system. This is a natural defense process but it puts the person under intolerable stress.

8-17/18

If the endocrine system (17/18) is found in the chain with the sex organs (8) there could be direct hormonal influence on the sex organs. If the person is a middle-aged woman, she may have a menopausal upset. If the individual is a man, he could have impotency. We see that 17/18 can associate with all organ numbers because each organ in itself has its own hormone balance. Each particular organ, cell and tissue and every nuclei in the body has its own 17/18 dichotomy. That is, each of these is composed of male and female energies, the male being pressure and the female being space; male being solidification and female being fragmentation; the male being fire and the female being water, to name a few examples. Therefore, we must understand that the whole existence of the body, from birth to death, is alive with male and female forces, while at the same time we understand that birth is a male principle and death is a female principle.

Mental Aspects

The mind (14), the brain (12) and the senses (15) are accentuated by the presence of 17/18 in an SAF chain. The brain (12) exudes a female characteristic. It possesses more energy that fragments and electrifies. The mind (14) is still more female and more beautiful in a sense that it can be completely cosmetic and filled with harmony. The mind (14) primarily induces the hypothalamus (15), a male-principled area that takes these female energies from the brain (12) and the mind (14) and flows thought-directed energies into the environment so that it can echo against pressures it finds for sensing. This technique – sensing – is extremely important for assessing the dragon disposition.

Because black body masses alone are the production of the mind and the brain, it seems necessary that these channels be used to sense out the dragons in the first place. The absolute Waterloo of doctors and medical practitioners all over the world is caused by the fact that the real traumas, the black body masses, are hidden from the view of the senses (15).

There is no way we can detect a dragon with the senses. We can't see it with our eyes because it is invisible. We can't hear it because it is soundless (sometimes we hear things, but it is all a dragon trick, an illusion); we can't smell it or touch it on this white body plane. Therefore, because scientists have had the inability to sense the black body masses with any usual apparatus, there is now a branch of "science" called psychiatry. However, in these psychiatrists' offices, and in the offices of most practitioners and nutritionists, the staff lacks the knowledge and the equipment (the SAF infrared sensor) to see these black body masses. They try all kinds of chemical approaches (chemicals are a male action in the sense of being condensive and not expansive), but ultimately, these don't treat the proper problem.

It seems that an orthodox health-oriented individual is doomed because he can't see the black body masses, and his doctor can't see the black body masses either. Adding male energy (drugs) to a body merely causes an even greater crush, condensation, confusion or cloudiness into the system and prevents anyone from ever being able to see black body masses.

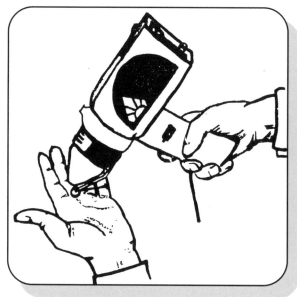

The infrared sensitizer in use.

The point is that the only way we can actually see black body masses is by using those channels of black body mass itself, the brain (12) and the mind (14). These are the only two avenues to detect a black body mass. These two female areas of the body are in the darkness and have the radiational capabilities of being able to, first of all, find the dragon and secondly, present it to the senses (15) for view.

12-14-15-17/18

The combination of the brain (12), the mind (14) and the hypothalamus (15), in coordination with the endocrine system (17/18), directs the spirituality of the individual to be able to focus enough attention and illumination mentally on these specific areas so that we can actually see what dragons are present.

While high technological advances in radiology have developed infrared scanners that view BBM (black body masses), scientists have yet to use it properly to hunt down dragons or traumas.

The SAF numerical chain that the author has been speaking of in great detail throughout this entire text is in itself a 17/18 hormone balance; it has male and female principles. Every action depicted to the left of the center of the chain is male and everything to the right is female. When we move from left to right of the chain, we are entering the past of the SAFent. We look at the past as a female principle because it is heaped in darkness; it has black body mass attached to it.

On the other hand, the condensation of these particles also produces the hormone balance in that black body masses themselves have male and female principles. There are male black body masses and there are female black body masses. The observation of these particular energies is simplistic. All we have to do is hook up to any galvanometer or electrical meter and bring forth (recall) traumatic experiences from the past and the pointer will move as the images and their energies drift by. This, of course, doesn't say whether the energies are male or female, but it does indicate that there has been some passage of energy through this human system. So, in this case, we must be very adept in the use of these machines to find and define the energies within the black body realms.

17/18-24

When the endocrine or hormone system (17/18) is connected with the lymph system (24) in an SAF chain, we observe that the enthusiastic production of trauma comes directly from the inducement of some drug or male principle that will knock out the person's ability to view black body masses.

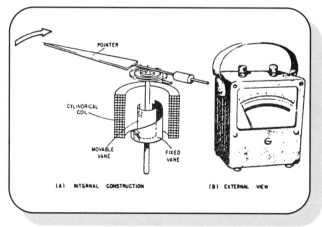

Those just beginning studies in self awareness and SAF might not understand the difference between white body light and black body light, or white body mass and black body mass.

Traumatic experiences from the past can be displayed on a meter as the energies go through a person's mind.

By studying SAF and running chains, SAFents will learn to make the distinction and will be able to see the past and know it is black body mass or black body radiation. As the electrical charge is discharged, the mental images become clearer. SAFents will find they have more energy and will be truly in the present time, which is white body mass and white body radiation.

White body light is the present time and is visible. Black body mass and black body radiation is the past time (invisible). Remember that 1% of energies are visible (white body mass) and 99% of energies are invisible (black body masses). If we are fifty years old, fifty years of life is steeped in black body mass while the exact moment of living, the present, is white body mass that we can confront.

This principle dictates that deep down the mind paths somewhere, a male dragon has been created by tremendous pressure or some kind of heavy impact, austere drug or operation. Or a female dragon was developed by the loss of a loved one or there was some disconnection from an energy source. These dragons must be confronted. They must be brought forward out of time and illuminated so they can be understood and controlled.

Physical Aspects

Because the endocrine system controls the entire look, feel and touch of the body, the energetic system of the body is tremendously dependent upon the endocrine program.

8-17/18

When the endocrine system (17/18) is associated with the sex organs (8), the individual may experience upsets in productivity and reproduction. The body is unable to copy itself in this position. Therefore, the person finds he is unable to reproduce cellular tissues to recreate the body. Because cells are dying and being sloughed off and then replaced moment to moment, any disruption may cause rapid aging. The actual creative mechanisms of the body in the physical sense can be thwarted and the body will lose creatine, a chemical substance (from the Greek *kreas* meaning "flesh"). Essentially, if he is unable to coordinate his hormone balance (17/18), it means he is losing flesh.

10-17/18

When an individual has the endocrine system (17/18) and the thyroid (10) together in his chain, then there is a chance that he may be overweight, swollen, heavy, and have much fatty tissue and water trapped in the body. The body structure is overstressed and the endocrine system doesn't want to cope with this.

1-17/18

If the endocrine system (17/18) is connected with the thymus (1), the SAFent has great difficulty protecting his body as a whole. Often, when this chain sequence goes into effect, the person's body can develop tumors. Lumps, bumps, tumors, and growths, especially around the thyroid, which is normally supposed to protect the body diagram and the genetically predicted shape.

1-10-17/18

The endocrine system (17/18), the thymus (1), and the thyroid (10) all in one chain sequence causes the worry that the protection of the body has been breached; the screens are down. If the kidneys (16) are in that same chain, then the body's ability to filter out poisons and to keep dragons at bay have also been reduced markedly. It is open season on this person. The dragons that are unable to see their own past very well may overwhelm this individual. The dragons may have memory loss and troubles with their own bodies because other dragons are so encrusted within them.

SAF Chains containing 1-10-17/18 and 1-10-16-17/18 in various configurations

1-10-17/18-19-20-21-22-24 ➤ overwhelm

3-4-5-6-11-1-10-17/18 ➤ past trauma

1-2-3-5-10-11-14-17/18 ➤ possible confusion

17/18-6-7-8-10-12-11-1 ➤ no worry

1-10-16-17/18-5-6-7-8-9 ➤ fear of overwhelm

2-3-5-6-7-1-10-16-17/18 ➤ overwhelming trauma

1-10-20-15-16-14-15-17/18 ➤ possible trauma

17/18-1-10-20-12-9-6-16 ➤ recent trauma

10-5-4-1-6-16-15-17/18 ➤ hysteria

The dragons are made up of black body masses and black body radiation that the host or victim can't see very well. These entities are invisible and they remain invisible. As long as they are invisible they are safe and they are happy. They don't want you to be able to see them. All they want to do is influence your life and find reminders (plays) for themselves so they can be fed, made stronger and happier. This is a positive activity for the dragons because they, too, want to live.

Therefore, we have to understand that for all energies and entities to remain in harmony there must be balance and coordination. When the 17/18 is coordinated and balanced, you can remain in total synchronization with all energies in the environment. You will finally get your reward of power, strength and total illumination.

19

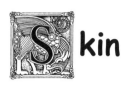
Skin

AT A GLANCE:
Emotion: Boredom
Condition: Demarcation

A protective encasement around the body, consisting of the dermis and its covering the epidermis, the skin is the largest organ of the human physical structure. The skin, in the 19th position in SAF, is the physical manifestation of the thymus (1). In other words, the skin is a solid crystalline shield that is in harmony with the protective outline of the thymus shield (1).

Emotion: Boredom

Few people understand the correlation of boredom with the skin. When individuals who complained of skin (19) troubles were questioned about their emotional states, it was found that there had been deep-set and chronic disillusionment or bored feelings with their present day circumstances. An individual's skin shouldn't be interesting or even visible; it should be invisible.

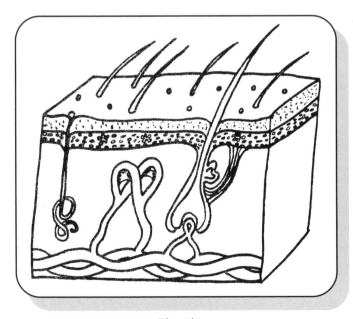

The Skin

As the skin (19) happens to be a harmonic of the thymus (1), it is a solidification of the thymus activity. The skin operates in a black light band that is itself infrared. Anything actually seen on the skin is crystallized matter – dead tissue. The reflected energies that hit the surface areas of the skin are the past content of energy systems that have gone more solid. The skin matrix itself is, and should be, invisible to the naked eye.

However, when poisons get lodged in the system, it causes warts, cysts, moles, pimples and things that can be seen. It causes the skin to become quite interesting. This, of course, is the opposite of boredom.

It seems that anything that affects the skin becomes chronic. Even with the advent of super creams to take away skin blemishes, the individual still has a constant battle on his hands. Once a person develops a certain kind of skin rash or skin problem, it can move into chronic states quite easily.

Condition: Demarcation

The skin draws the line for the existence of one entity as opposed to another. As mentioned, the skin itself is an invisible entity. Therefore, it is impossible to tell when one entity is crossing the boundary line of another.

This confuses many people because the skin surface has its own tangible, reliable sense, the sense of touch. In reality, that sense of touch can be expanded out for several miles. We can have what is called expanded tactile sense that allows us to perceive feelings from great distances. In a sense, this is the outreach of the skin itself and allows us to have the ability to contact other entities and zones of existence. The skin draws a specific boundary line; it acts as a border.

On the planetary level, all countries have borders. Depending on the country, you can either cross easily or you can be delayed for hours or days. In some parts of the world, all you have to do is acknowledge the fact that the border exists, nod to the guard and move across the line to the next country.

The pervasion of energies (border crossings) into the body from the environment is quite easy as well. The body is constantly and chronically being entered by outside forces. Examples would be the gaseous atmosphere that mixes the liquid condensation of humidity and dissolves the solids that float in the air, the water we drink, the food we ingest, the bugs, toxins and other poisons crossing the boundary lines of the skin. Because of all this, you may consider the skin to be in a state of overwhelm. The skin itself is an important matrix that helps decide whether or not an entity or energy should be pulled in closer to the core of the body or pushed out toward the perimeter. This is the ultimate responsibility of the thymus (1) and the thyroid (10).

Mental Aspects

The feature of number 19, when considering SAF numerical chain sequences, is that your body must be guarded from a state of overwhelm. Obviously, if the inner body were exposed to the cruel exterior environment, the amount of pressure would be immense. If you were to peel the outer epidermis off and expose the interior to the outside environment, the amount of energy impressions that would reach inside the body would be too much to bear. You would go into a state of shock and may not survive. Such is the case with burn victims. So the skin acts as that protective shell that stops or slows down outside energies from moving into the body.

Protections on mental and spiritual levels are connected as well. SAF numeric chains foretell that the mind is constantly aware of its perimeter and is watchful to maintain its separation from other individuals. A person must mentally draw the line in his mind and be able to coordinate his activities within the boundaries of his own existence.

15-19

Many times a person's energies breach another's boundaries. When the hypothalamus (15) and the skin (19) are connected in a SAF chain producing the 15-19 sequence, it indicates that energies within one person's body may have intersected with another. Many times it is a conclusion of the SAF Monitor observing such a combination that someone has crossed over his SAFent's boundary and has not yet left; the interloper is still in there with him. This enmeshing occurs often so it is important that each person doing self awareness work fill out his or her own questionnaire to reduce the risk of producing a combined chain.

19-22

When the parathyroid (22) is connected with the skin (19), there may have developed a specific encrustation of energy within another person's mind, brought about by a fit of anger.

15-19 Combinations in an SAF numerical chain

15-16-17/18-19-4-5-10-20-23-9 ➤ intermittent crossover

10-16-20-4-5-8-15-19 ➤ full possession

19-20-4-5-8-1-15 ➤ entity left (numbers reversed)

4-10-5-19-15-20-17/18-16-3-12 ➤ entity tries to escape

15-14-4-5-6-20-8-10-19 ➤ entity intrusion

10-19-8-6-12-15-16-20-17/18-4 ➤ entity lost

The above combinations indicate the energies in one person's body may have intersected with that of another person.

Few people realize that becoming angry with another person, or pressing any negative energy towards another, causes particles of your own energies to breach the other's mental skin or demarcation line, thereby endowing that person with more opposing energy. It seems the successful operation of pacifism is the conservation of energy. When we become very angry with another individual, we merely impress an energy pattern in that other person's system that gives the other more energy and power to oppose us.

With this view in mind, it is nonsensical to create any situation that is of an attack nature. War and any kind of aggressive action would seem to only feed the other side.

The sequence 19-22 doesn't necessarily designate a war-like individual. This person has experienced the encrustation of dragons from other areas that could be toxins, pollutants, minerals and things of this nature. Poisons in the body may certainly create the sudden manifestation of 19-22 in an SAF chain that appear as some abrasion, lump, bump, callous, corn or roughened area of the skin. This gives us the idea that there has been some violation of territory on a mental basis. The aggression doesn't necessarily have to be on a physical level. Be aware that when mental energy impresses itself into the body, it can create a physical reaction.

Physical Aspects

Perhaps the most fascinating part of the SAF project is the use of the SAF Infrared Sensor. This particular sensitizing machine is programmed into the high-tech mathematical matrix that utilizes the 23 organ and gland systems. In the 1970s it had been theorized that the actual electric and magnetic nature of the symptoms, diseases and traumas of an individual could be tracked. This led to the understanding that there were definite entities involved for each specific disease syndrome. These entities, later called dragons, have affinity for particular gland systems and create specific diseases such as diabetes, arthritis, cancer and all the known maladies of mankind. Different machinery was used in experiments and ultimately the infrared sensing device was incorporated. It used a two-dimensional flat plane for scanning, which gave SAF practitioners a view of the precise symmetry of energy patterns in the body. The program was actually interfacing with the demarcation areas of the skin and looking inside the body. It was able to read exactly which organ systems were heating up and which were cooling down. By observing these particular patterns of energy (hot glands/organs and cold glands/organs), we could see that there was a specific overload of energy or toxins in specific areas of the body.

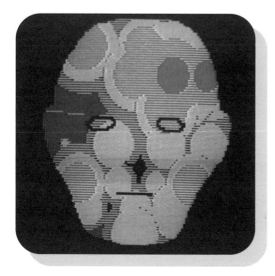

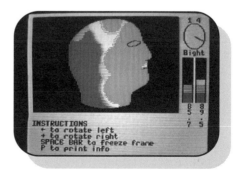

Left, Infrared face picture. Above, 3-D infrared image. Templates of the human body were designed to be used in a vast array of therapies such as chiropractic, iridology, and symptomatology. These infrared temperature readings are linked to the SAF mathematical matrix.

The original two dimensional scanning program gave rise to the creation of a three-dimensional scanning technique. Venting sites were mapped and energy coordinates were cataloged. Infrared proves the theory that energies can know and intersect with other energies and be translated.

The solution to understanding the physical anomalistic manifestations of the skin – rashes, pimples, boils, tumors and all the irregularities that cause the skin to become more visible and less boring – are easily observed by either scanning with the infrared sensitizing equipment or completing a questionnaire.

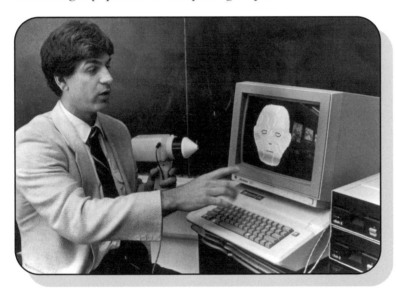

Joseph R. Scogna, Jr. explains the use of infrared and the computer, 1986. Scogna adapted the infrared sensor to allow it to interface with the SAF mathematical matrix.

19-20

Problems of the skin are more observable when the pancreas (20) is connected with the skin (19) in a numerical chain. This particular sequence is called psoriasis. It represents that psoriatic entry point where a dragon has penetrated.

The toxins and poisons that desire entrance won't be allowed in when the body is aware of their actual natures. But because dragons hide in black body mass and black body radiation, in what is considered dark light or invisible light, no one can see them. They have a vested interest in creating "holes" in the skin so they can enter. It is theorized by the author (and is by practical nature a useable theory) that all skin manifestations are merely entry holes for enterprising dragons to develop or spawn energies more compatible with their own natures.

SAF Chains and 19-20 Configurations

<u>19-20</u>-1-2-5-7-9-10-15 ➤ red patches

1-2-5-7-9-10-15-<u>19-20</u> ➤ chronic red patches

1-2-5-7-<u>19-20</u>-9-10-15 ➤ worried about red patches

<u>19</u>-2-5-7-10-15-9-1-<u>20</u> ➤ possible red patches

<u>20</u>-1-2-5-7-10-15-9-<u>19</u> ➤ no red patches

1-2-<u>19</u>-5-7-10-<u>20</u>- 9-15 ➤ intermittent red patches

1-<u>20</u>-2-5-7-10-9-<u>19</u>-15 ➤ red patches leaving

1-2-5-<u>20-19</u>-7-10-9-15 ➤ stuck red patches

1-19

When the thymus (1) connects with the skin (19), we see the extent of pressure brought to bear upon the skin's surfaces; the individual has been inundated by toxins to the point that he is losing his border integrity. This (1-19) situation involves calor (heat), dolar (pain), rubar (redness) and tumor (swelling). These four reactions are able to track when a dragon has attacked the body. The action of these particular dragons is powerful enough to escape detection by the naked eye. In other words, you can't see a dragon actually performing, but you certainly can see its effects. As a result, many people have the mistaken impression that the skin rash, boil or pimple or whatever they do see sitting there is the dragon, so they attack what they <u>think</u> is the dragon. They apply creams, balms or herbs hoping to vanquish it. There is even a salve called "dragon balm." However, the action of putting a topical cream on an area infested with a poison or toxin merely pushes the substances and the dragon deeper inside the body. The important thing to do is to express the poison back outside the body.

We must be sure to recognize that any kind of manifestation in visible light form is the spawn of the actual dragon, created out of black body light or black body radiation. The real entities that are working their magic against the body are invisible.

20

ancreas/

olar Plexus

At number 20, the pancreas/solar plexus is special because human beings depend on this complex for balance. The pancreas allows us to decide between substances in the environment. In this way, toxins and poisons, vermin, parasites, pests and other kinds of creatures not desirable to the body are pressed out, and anything usable that can become part of the body in a productive way will be accepted inside the system.

The pancreas is loaded with enzymes that help in the digestion of fats, minerals and sugars. If in proper working condition, we depend on it to keep us balanced in the presence of all activity.

The solar plexus is the nerve center that balances the nervous system. It is directly connected to the earth's center of gravity. From the very moment a baby is born, we can see it flail its arms as it struggles to maintain its balance. By using the exact center of gravity of the body, which is the solar plexus, we learn to maintain stability in the presence of all stimuli from the environment.

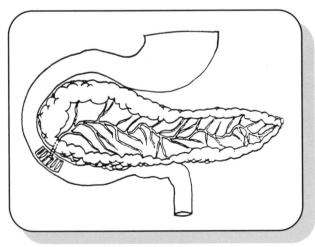

The Pancreas

No matter which way we are pushed or shoved, we can regain our balance by observing this contact between the solar plexus and the earth's solar plexus, the very epicenter of the earth itself. This balancing is a practical action for the entire body, and with the help of the pancreas, it is centered in electrical charges of a positive and negative nature.

In chemistry, this is called pH (the potential of Hydrogen), or the acid-basic balance. This is maintained quite readily by the pancreas and the pancreatic juices, for one of its purposes is to sustain the equilibrium of energy in the body by controlling the sugar balance with two hormones called glucagon and insulin. So, if you have any disharmony of these hormones, the homeostasis of the body will be thrown off and you will feel off center.

Emotion: Laughter

People who complained of loss of balance, dizziness, vertigo, low energy, etc. were found to have the number 20 in the lead portion of their chains.

The loss of balance is directly associated with the person's inability to maintain or direct the energy conditions of the body.

Laughter is a good measure of a deficiency of balance because it is part of the solar plexus mechanism of discharging unwanted energies in the body. It is amazing to observe and detect the actual discharge processes by monitoring the way people laugh. Each laugh has a distinctive way of discharging toxins from the system. It is true that individuals who don't laugh are very ill. At the same time, laughter has to be precise and it has to explode or discharge toxins of all sorts in an extremely wide variety of subjects, or else different poisons that have been encrusted into a person's body will stay there.

It is part of the life continuum that mind energy in connection with spiritual energy produces a magnetic and electric attraction for toxins in the environment. If you have particular problems, or can't figure out enough patterns of energy to become productive, then you will actually call in specific toxins from your environment. In other words, if you are loaded with poison, such as parasites, worms, bacteria or viruses, they were brought to the body because you were into a behavioral pattern that acted like an antenna in the body to attract these poisons. The poisons and solid matter are the last step in the creation chain of interference with someone's energy.

So it is herein explained that if a person doesn't laugh – and laugh correctly – these poisons can't be discharged from his body and he will rapidly fester and die a painful death. There are experts on the subject of laughter, and authors with ideas on how to maintain a happy existence. Part of this happiness necessitates the action of laughing.

A person can be found out to be a charlatan in his laughing attitude. Just because you laugh doesn't mean you are getting rid of toxins or discharging energy. Your laugh may be merely a social gesture. A placating laugh is not therapeutic. Such a laugh is from the throat.

We must laugh from the solar plexus, which is beneath the diaphragm, to discharge poison from the body. The discharges are explosive. The interfering energies of dragons that have been compressed into the system need to be exploded out of the body. If you merely laugh from the chest, throat, or nose, or if you snicker, titter, twitter, chuckle, or carry on in any way the toxins will remain inside the body. When a person tries to laugh, his laughter can truncate a dragon, chopping it off at the top and leaving

167

a substantial portion of the bottom. To reiterate it is essential for a proper release that you follow the correct laughing procedure, and experiences an actual "belly laugh."

How do we learn to laugh correctly? The only way to create a correct laugh is by understanding the principle. When we make the connection between actions of the cause of the dragon and the actions of the effect of the dragon, then we can make the proper laughing reaction.

What is the mechanism of laughter? When we see something that causes us to laugh, what exactly is occurring? How do we connect with the dragon when we see someone fall and hurt himself? That action, of course, is a replay of a certain trauma of the observing individual. The reason the observer laughs is because he is replaying his own trauma. The dragon that lurks within a person's mind is a mental image of he himself falling. All the jokes and stories that cause others to laugh, and the hysterical movie scenes are part of the invisible dragon content. The only reason a person laughs is because a connection to the dark side has been touched upon and brought into the visible light, into white body light. Something has come to the senses that used to be invisible. It was harbored in black body light for a long time. Making this connection causes an electrical surge that actually explodes a piece of the dragon. To edit a dragon, to delete the electrical charge of it from your existence, you need to see all of it. One of the "windows" into the dragon may be the peculiar aspect of the trauma that is brought into view, the one that causes you to laugh.

In the final analysis, we must differentiate a courtesy laugh from the electrical discharge laugh, which occurs when a piece of black body light is thrust into the visible light spectrum.

Condition: Location

We should routinely look for the number 20 within all numerical chains because 20 connects with many other numbers to produce a variety of traumatic sources and content. Number 20 is typical of an individual who has lost his ability to locate himself. The question "Where am I?" is made clear when the number 20 is in a numerical chain sequence.

You may know where you are consciously, but depending on where the number 20 is in the chain, and with which numbers it is connected, it may indicate that certain organs and organ functions are lost inside the body or mind. In other words, the SAFent doesn't have to be lost, but one or several of his organs could be. If they are lost as to their location, they are certainly lost to their correct balance and function.

6-20

If, for example, the liver (6) is connected to the pancreas (20), this is an indication that an individual's liver is either too acid or too basic. In other words, it is losing its location frequency because it is vibrating with too much toxin or poison, and not enough of its own interstitial integrity.

2-20

When the number 20 is connected to the heart (2), it shows that the SAFent has lost a person or entity, something that produced much heat for him in the past, and which has now been subtracted from his life.

This information is extremely important, for it creates an effective dragon and (as was explained previously) this particular dragon is of a <u>female</u> nature, for it has created a <u>loss</u> in the system.

These losses are capable of moving from the invisible or dark light spectrum into the white light spectrum, causing the individual specific damage to the heart muscle. Although it is wholly a mental phenomenon associated with the viewpoint that the individual has lost at life, it certainly has a specific effect on the human system - a net energy loss. When an individual is connected with another, their energies co-mingle; when the partner is lost, the remaining person will find himself in a position of still relying on energy factors that were peculiar to the lost person. This causes a feeling of groping by the electrical mechanisms in the body. As this "nervous" system tries to replenish the lost energies from the individual who is gone, the body will experience a good deal of symptomatology.

Mental Aspects

SAFents who present the number 20 in numerical chains have definite location problems, exhibiting an increased sense of dispersion and confusion. The real problem stems from environmental dragons. Traumas that have occurred in specific locations and have collected the energy of their surroundings (grass, trees, roads, cars, buildings, mountains, sky, atmosphere, etc.) have caused a black body mass to occur with an image of a location where the individual used to be.

13-20

When the adrenal glands (13) is with the pancreas (20) in an SAF chain, then the individual may have difficulty eliminating the electrical charge connected with a certain area in which he used to live. The energies (patterns of motion) from that former location may have caused his molecular structure to go into phase with those same energies. When we relocate to a new home, we have to shift the energies to the new location. Because people in modern day society are more transient than ever before, this particular quirk shows up frequently. The 13-20 is called homesickness and depression. It occurs because of a lost ability to track the energies of the present surroundings.

Another unusual phenomenon that occurs is the attraction of energy from the particular location and time of our birth. Suppose it was Philadelphia on November 3rd, 1962 at 3 AM. Our energies have been primed or initialized by that precise time and place. If we are not sure where or when we were born, or how we came into this world, we will have a constant subliminal dispersion about our environment. It is essential to de-confuse an individual by locating him. It is necessary to edit out the time and location dragons of environmental pasts so the SAFent is free to be in the present.

10-20

When the thyroid (10) connects with the pancreas (20), the individual may be in a very confused situation. The 10-20 individual may have difficulty prioritizing activities, or knowing what is important. He has trouble being in the right place at the right time. Such a person is represented as negligent or irresponsible about his duties or his activities. He should spend more time developing an awareness of what his true goals and purposes are in life, so he can be in the right place at the right time.

1-20

Another interesting combination occurs when the thymus (1) associates with the pancreas (20); this particular mathematical string signifies frustration. It is a frustration of energy not completed, such as programs and ideas that have not come to fruition. The 1-20 individual is often thwarted, even though he may exhibit the sensation of energies nearly coming into being.

This occurs often in individuals who have almost finished a project or who have almost finished a trip. It is called the "trip end," when energies (ideas, plans, formats) are almost in completion and the electrical friction and the vibration and power of these two ideas (completing but yet not completed) causes such a rash of electrical stimulation in the system that the person becomes super sensitized and loses his ability to remain calm and collected.

SAF Chains and 1-20 Sequences

1-20-22-24-2-8-10-12-14 ➤ frustration

22-24-2-8-10-12-14-1-20 ➤ frustrated

1-2-4-8-10-22-12-24-20 ➤ probably frustration

20-12-2-4-8-10-22-24-1 ➤ relief (orgasm)

2-4-6-10-8-1-20-22-24-12-14-15 ➤ temptation

2-4-1-5-6-20-22-24-12 ➤ chronic temptation

2-4-20-5-6-1-22-24-12 ➤ chronic orgasm

2-4-5-6-20-1-10-15-17/18-12 ➤ worried about orgasms

Physical Aspects

The physical aspects of the pancreatic insufficiencies or toxicity rely on the ability of the solar plexus to maintain balance and harmony within the system. The energies of the body may dip or subside as there are shifts and changes between the two hormones glucagon and insulin. There may be either an increase of power or there may be a sharp and sudden decrease during which the SAFent feels drained.

Many modern day nutritional scientists have run with the idea that hypoglycemia can be applied to individuals who exhibit this sudden change or drop in energy. However, the hypoglycemic condition can be caused by frustration, the loss of a loved one, irresponsibility, homesickness and many other conditions that disconnect the person's power supply, causing him to lose energy in a physiological or psychological way.

Other researchers contend that their work is directed at cerebral or stress allergies. Stress allergies are processed by the body, and the cross connection of power, which is the matrix of the genetic machines in response to the present day white body light system, causes the physical body to be sapped momentarily of strength. This is a genuine problem, but one solved by SAF chain discovery. Because these dragons have friends, we need to discover the whole mechanism, not just part of it.

1-20

When an individual has a thymus (1) and pancreas (20) in his chain, he may develop what is called chancre. Ulcers, ulceration sores and spots on the body result from toxins that have built up to such an extent that there is a burning or an incineration of tissues. This may be brought about by the introduction of some energy or poison into the system, but in many cases it is a direct phenomenon of sexual perversity. The perversion comes about when the body reacts to the insertion of energies (diagrams and forms of sex) with human beings, animals or objects. As a human person tries to intersect his energies (life-stream continuity) or reproduces energies (his own) in a variety of animal, vegetable and mineral substances on the planet, he finds that only one species can actually reproduce his species correctly. A man needs a woman to reproduce the biophysical schema of the genes. Sexual activity is a precision act, even though many times the perpetrators are unschooled at the process. When an individual deviates from the protocol for sexual behavior, the acid-basic balance is disturbed and acid conditions begin to build up. The thymus gland (1) and the pancreas (20) or solar plexus location have difficulty handling the scenario of the geometric patterns created by erratic resonant frequencies that can bounce back and forth between bodies during sex.

The human body can certainly handle normal sexual contact, but when a person starts to introduce objects, animals and other paraphernalia into the system, the electrical natures that coexist between these particular objects creates a resonance that can create specific sores and ulcers in the body. The body may not be able to digest or absorb this kind of energy (dissimilar objects). It has no genetic program plate or blueprint to understand anything but another similar body, so it puts the energy (molecules of the dissimilar substance or person) on hold near the skin.

1-16-19-20

Many times when the thymus (1), the kidneys (16) and the skin (19) are seen with the pancreas (20) in a chain, it indicates that there is a presence of genetically or recently (present time) transmitted gonorrhea, syphilis, herpes or other venereal conditions. If the hypothalamus (15) and the endocrine system (17/18) are added to this same chain sequence, then we may have the right to fear the development of AIDS. If the person has this same unfortunate chain sequence containing the adrenals (13), he may have compromised his immune system even further. He may be at the point where the particular energies (people, places and events) are in such an uproar that they are unable to complete the entire diagram of energy (proper sex act to completion).

SAF Chains and 1-16-19-20 Combinations:

1-16-19-20-4-12-8-22-17/18-14 ➤ venereal disease

8-22-14-17/18-6-16-20-1-19 ➤ genetic venereal disease

14-17/18-20-16-19-1-8-24 ➤ worried about venereal disease

1-15-16-20-8-14-17/18-22-19-24 ➤ chronic venereal disease

16-20-17/18-14-8-2-1-10-15-19 ➤ possible venereal disease

2-10-13-1-16-15-19-20-22-17/18 ➤ AIDS

22-1-10-13-16-15-12-9-8-14-17/18-19-20 ➤ venereal entities (dragons)

19-20

When the skin (19) is associated with the pancreas (20), this is another indication that toxins and poisons may be stuck on the skin trying to gain entrance to the body. The person may have rashes, pimples, sores and other skin phenomena. This can indicate that the black body masses and radiation toxins, those that endemically belong to dragons of the deep past, are influencing the present and trying to work their way into the system, destroying the present time body matrix.

13-20

If the adrenal glands (13) and the pancreas (20) are found in a chain, the person may have chronic hypoglycemia. His energies may be at a low ebb. This occurs when the dramatic content of dragon sequences have entered the system and lie across the person's energies in such a way that he is not able to recover his energy (life) without drastic measures. With pancreatic insufficiency, the person may have sharp drops in energy but then regain his energy, whereas with a 13-20 sequence, he may be chronically tired and exhausted.

SAF Chains and 13-20 combinations

13-20-14-15-17/18-2-10-4-22 ➤ loss of location

20-10-4-22-14-15-17/18-13-20 ➤ lost connection

20-10-4-22-13-20-14-15-17/18-1 ➤ lost love

13-15-14-16-17/18-2-10-4-22-20 ➤ possible losses

20-15-14-16-17/18-2-10-4-22-13 ➤ no loss

2-4-10-22-20-13-15-16-8-24 ➤ coping

2-4-20-5-13-15-16-8-24 ➤ chronic cope

7-8-9-4-10-16-8-20-13 ➤ no organization

21

osterior Pituitary

AT A GLANCE:
Emotion: Grief
Condition: Liquification

The 21st gland in the SAF sequence is the posterior pituitary, which lies directly behind the anterior pituitary and is connected to the hypophyseal stalk. The action of the posterior pituitary is specific in the creation of lactating hormones that control the milk production in postpartum females and the release of the unfertilized egg in the ovary. The posterior pituitary also releases anti-diuretic hormones when needed to control the fluid balance or the fluid permeability in the membranes of the human body. This gland controls the actual swelling or water secretion in the body.

Emotion: Grief

Many SAFents with number 21 appearing first in the SAF chains, complained of great losses. When the SAF Monitor sees the number 21, he understands that losses and degradations have occurred where energy (people, places, things, and businesses) has been pulled away from the SAFent. It is significant to note that the number (21), therefore, seems to have a primarily female bent. Number (21) controls a losing or expanding nature. It is concerned with space (mind -14) and with the ability of the body to maintain or reproduce new energies out of old energies (sex organs - 8). The losses found in the physical system are caused primarily by deficiencies. These deficiencies are losses of pressure concerning every circumstance.

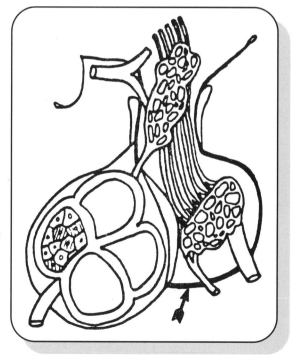

The Posterior Pituitary

When we lose pressure, objects, people and places, we find we are in the untenable position of having energies that we need desperately (any object, person, place, thing) being stolen away from us. A mythological story exemplifies this scenario. Tantalus, a Greek God, was tied upside down in Hades and tantalized. Food and drink were held out to him, but every time he reached out they were pulled back from his grasp. Number 21 exemplifies this kind of frustration, but it is a frustration that can be balanced to cause pleasant sensation. The winning or the gaining of something pleasurable depends on movements towards the pressure end of the scale. The numbers that are lower in the scale, such as 1, 2, 3, or 4, show pressurization. The numbers that are higher on the scale, such as 20, 21, 22, 23, or 24, indicate space. As we move higher on the scale, we notice more losses of pressure and more gains of space. If we wanted to pressurize number 21, we would move toward the pancreas (20). This slight increase of pressure causes the grief or loss (crying) (21) to turn to laughter (20). Laughter ensues because we have regained some pressure.

This can be easily demonstrated. When a young child cries because he has lost a plaything, replacing it with another plaything can immediately cause him to laugh again. He giggles because he has gotten another pressure to replace the loss of the previous pressure. All humans whether babies, adolescents, mature individuals or old persons, need to have the correct amount of pressure to create pleasure. On the other hand, too much pressure or too much stress creates the sensation of gain that may be too much to bear, which creates a condition of overwhelm. The opposite of this is, of course, the number (21), which guards the portal of loss. People try desperately to avoid losses at all costs.

Condition: Liquification

The appearance of the number (21) suggests difficulty controlling water balance.

2-21

When the heart (2) and the pituitary (21) present themselves together in an SAF chain, the individual may have swelling and edema. This swelling occurs because the person is trying to hold on to as much conductant as he can to produce pressure and charge. When losing the water content of the body, the person doesn't need as much conductant. In fact, he needs more insulation. Things happen too fast for some people and they dump water to escape the charge. When we start to swell with water, things are happening too slowly.

When projects and plans are not resolving fast enough, bodies begin to swell up with water so that more conductivity can take place. As the pace of things begins to move more rapidly, the water is dumped.

SAF Chains and 2-21 combinations
2-21-23-24-16-1-5-4-10 ➤ lost love
2-4-1-6-5-21-16-23-20 ➤ possible loss
21-24-7-9-8-20-2 ➤ no loss of love
1-4-6-10-21-2-5-9-24 ➤ worried about losing love

Mental Aspects

The number 21 indicates the loss of energy (ideas, plans and dreams). There may be several aspects to the losses, but they involve the disconnection of our ability to observe our own mental experiences (memory) in relation to the present day situation. Our primary loss is the inability to rectify what has happened to us in the past (which is invisible as it lies in black body mass), as opposed to what is happening to us in the present (visible, white body masses), or what will happen to us in the future (invisible, black body mass). If we can't rectify or connect these ideas, then our power is reduced proportionately. The more we can rectify our past with our present, the more powerful we become for the future, because the past is where all the energy patterns (existence patterns) are stored. It is these energy patterns, the actual outline or blueprint that give us power. Nothing else.

14-21

When the mind (14) is found with the posterior pituitary (21) in an SAF chain, the individual may have lost some of his memory.

1-14-21

If the thymus (1) is in the vicinity, it indicates how much memory is lost. Thymus (1) indicates it is the highest amount that could be lost. It is a matter of how close in proximity the numbers are in a numerical chain that gives an idea of just how severe is the memory loss.

1-14-17/18-21

If, in the previous same chain (1-14-21) the individual also exhibits the endocrine system (17/18), it is important to note that the memory loss is due to some presence and organization of dragon systems. There may be a trauma overlaid between the person's conscious mind and the person's unconscious mind, blocking white body masses from being able to intercept and rectify black body masses of the past. Therefore the individual effectively has his energy (memory banks) cut from him.

15-21

When the hypothalamus (15) and the posterior pituitary (21) are present together in a chain, this indicates that the person is trying to sense, connect with and rectify energy mates (lovers) from the past through the sexual radar, which is part of the pineal body's system.

SAF chains and 1-14-17/18-21 Combinations

1-14-17/18-21-22-24 ➤ Acute memory loss

2-3-6-10-13-1-14-17/18-21 ➤ Chronic Memory loss

2-10-1-14-17/18-21-22-24 ➤ Alzheimer's disease

1-2-10-14-17/18-22-24-21 ➤ Possible memory block

21-2-10-17/18-14-22-24-1 ➤ Minimal memory loss

14-21-5-17/18-2-1-24 ➤ Intermittent memory loss

17/18-2-1-21-5-22-14 ➤ Functional memory

21-17/18-14-1-7-9-10 ➤ Perceptive

Physical Aspects

It has already been explained that the posterior pituitary has the capability of containing water in the system, so a person may have swelling or a physical effect of energy being lost in the system. One of the worst sicknesses of mankind – diabetes insipidus – comes about when the anti-diuretic hormone is deficient, causing the loss of great amounts of urine and excessive thirst. The body's water is not able to cleanse toxins from the system through the lymph tract (24). We must ensure there is a proper mineral balance to consistently cause the physical side of the number 21 to have a proper action of gain and loss.

If the posterior pituitary (21) causes too much loss in the system, the SAFent may be in the position of experiencing too much sensation. He may have dizziness, nausea, vomiting, and just errant electrical charges that cause uncomfortable sensations in the body. On the other hand, if the system is overloaded with pressure and the body can't control the water balance to disallow pressure buildup in the system, he may have pain and pressure. The pain will be in various areas of the body, but mostly in the joints and in the muscles of the lower back. The body is not able to fight off pressure if it can't control water balance in the system, for the water is used as the primary conductor of electric charge.

If the water in the body is dirty and filled with poisonous toxins, chemicals, drugs, and unwanted minerals, then the system will have a very erratic electrical pattern. For this reason, the body will often opt to create fatty substances as a protection or insulation, or choose to dump water in the body to rid itself of some of these toxins. One of the most effective ways to rid a body of toxins is by exercise and sweat. As sweat moves off the body it carries the dragon's eggs (noxious wastes) with it.

22

arathyroid Gland

AT A GLANCE:
Emotion: Anger
Condition: Experience

The parathyroid gland is strongly resilient to radiation and has been assigned number 22. The gland creates a visible shield, in the form of calcium, to ward off radiant forces. The balancing hormones for calcium in the physical body are calcitonin and parathormone, and between these two hormones, the regulation of calcium is predictable. However, the intrinsic study of energy and radiant sources in and around the body demands that we know the precise endocrine duties of the parathyroid gland. The parathyroid gland acts as an invincible third shield against radiation. The first shield is the thymus (1), the second is the thyroid (10), and the third is the parathyroid (22).

The parathyroid shields the body against radiation by creating calcium deposits. The calcium precipitant is equivalent to one drop of experience in the presence of radiation, electricity and excess pressure. The amount of calcium produced depends on the exact amount of pressure brought to bear on the recording systems of the body, mind and spirit.

In a very real sense, the energies of the individual, as he is acting throughout life, are inscribed in his system; the action of the parathyroid helps to produce the skeletal structure. The axial and the appendicular skeletal systems are merely outreaches of experience in the body.

A human baby starts life with very little calcium in his body (calcium is the lightest metal on the planet Earth). As the baby grows and experiences life, calcium precipitates into the bones. This calcium is

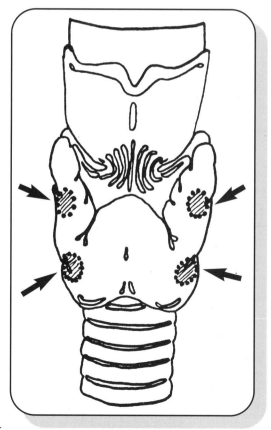

The Parathyroid Gland

absorbed and reduced into mental and spiritual experiences and then constantly replaced by new calcium as a daily routine. These actions occur hourly, microsecond by microsecond. This process activates the learning and the experiential memory banks of the body.

Emotion: Anger

A person will be in an angry symptom pattern when the number 22 appears in the forefront of the numerical chain. Anger develops when an individual refuses to change his idea or opinion about a certain circumstance or scenario.

Anger follows the experiential tracks of the memory recordings for a human being because anger is considered a solidification or frozen edifice in space. The precipitate of calcium, which is a memory experience, is in itself without opposition, and won't tolerate any other viewpoint. Therefore, a mental picture mirrors the exact emotional pattern of anger, which disregards all other ideas, programs, purposes and viewpoints other than its own.

10-22

When the thyroid (10) is in the same numerical chain as the parathyroid (22), then we see the exact energy (pattern) sequence of the spine. The spine is the principle mechanism for the motor operations of a human being. It is the actual experience track or memory staff, which coordinates and structures much of the electrical output for the brain and the mind throughout the nervous system, to create emotional experiences regulated by the glands and organs of the body. In other words, the spine acts as a conducting post for all the whims, desires and dreams of an individual. Any degradation of the spine indicates that certain areas are being over-pressurized or under-pressurized by either high acid or high alkaline conditions.

Specific levels of energy (physical input versus output) are received by the body. These messages are tracked by the intensity of pressure in the environment so that the memory recordings being made can be the exact depth or intensity. The human being records experience and energy (happenings in the environment and in the body) in much the same way as we would record an idea, a thought or a program on magnetic tape. The energy recordings etched onto the magnetic tape cause a mark to appear of a certain depth and design.

By having the precise groove of a person's experience of a certain depth and design, we are able to have the correct emotional response. If this groove is too deep, we will have a traumatic experience; this is considered toxicity. If the groove of experience is too light, then we will have a deficiency. With a deficiency, there is also a trauma because we have lost the amount of pressure necessary to perceive the true circumstances surrounding us.

Condition: Experience

As mentioned above, experience is the mark of the action to which we are exposed. The experience track is developed by a precipitation of calcium with etchings or grooves in it that give the proper scenario for replay. The body takes this particular calcium experience track and records it in each cell as the calcium is dissolved and replaced for a new set of experience. The spine is a particular energy post that governs and coordinates experiences and emotions throughout all the glands and organs in the system.

As we look at the entire system of a human being, we realize the experiences of a human being are of paramount importance to his survival. The way we acquire knowledge and understanding is directly parallel to this experience process. Knowledge, in coordination with mental activities, awareness and understanding, and with spiritual activities, works in harmony with the proper experiences necessary to coordinate our activity toward total survival (immortality).

1-22

When the thymus gland (1) is found with the parathyroid gland (22) in the same SAF chain, then the individual may experience the inability to protect himself. It shows that poisons and toxins from the environment are encroaching on his system and may be stealing away the ability to re-contact his past experiences for survival actions in the present.

Mental Aspects

We have to imagine the parathyroid (22) along with the experiential activities of the body, as a shield or wall. As the thymus (1) is the invisible, electronic shield and the thyroid (10) is that physical or flesh shield, then the parathyroid (22) is the structural shield, the shield that protects the <u>core</u> of the individual. No wonder he becomes angry! He certainly doesn't want any other person entering, disturbing or invading the core of his being. The number 22 is the last shield of a person's inner self, and if this number <u>does</u> appear in the SAF numerical chain, it indicates that the person's core essence is being encroached upon, invaded.

14-22

When the mind (14) and the parathyroid (22) present themselves, the person may be exhibiting a complete frustration or anger with the amount of attack or barrage of mental poisons that are affecting him. He is conceptually angry at all the troubles that are befalling him and he is not coping with any of them. It is important to watch the drift of these numbers so we can understand just how much effect the troubles or confrontations are having on this person's existence. As far as understanding the flow or drift of the numbers in numerical chain sequences, we can see the actual movement of a particular upset as successive scans are taken or additional questionnaires are evaluated.

2-22

When the heart (2) is connected to the parathyroid (22), there is an alert or a signal in the numerical chain indicating that the individual is dissatisfied or disgruntled with his connections with friends or loved ones. This person may be ripe for a separation or divorce. He has difficulty connecting the proper channels of information with his loved ones and partners because he is unable to communicate with them properly.

It can be difficult for us to communicate with any other individual because we each have our very own experience tracks. As one person experiences an incident in the environment, another person may do so in an opposite way. Each would possess a completely different experience of the same occurrence. If we don't obtain the ability to change our mind or viewpoint and direct our own experiences, or if we are not able to take on the experiences of another person, then we will certainly develop a 2-22 sequence. This particular sequence in a chain, (2-22), is very detrimental for any individual who is trying to maintain a relationship.

2-20

To expound on the above scenario (2-22) two pressure-steps farther, to heart (2) and pancreas (20), we have a sequence that is separation, loss of friend, lover or ally. So, a 2-22 is a very important pre-signal to an elementary, detrimental characteristic of humankind, which is the inability to communicate effectively with loved ones or partners. The invasion of a friend can't be a productive experience if these two numbers (2-22) are "hot."

SAF Chains and 2-22 Combinations

2-22-1-10-12-15-17/18-14-24 ➤ Argument

1-10-12-15-17/18-14-24-2-22 ➤ Suppressed Argument

2-1-10-12-15-17/18-14-24-22 ➤ Possible Conflict

22-1-10-12-15-17/18-14-24-2 ➤ No Contest

1-10-12-15-2-22-14-24-17/18 ➤ Worried About Fighting

1-10-12-15-22-2-14-17/18-5 ➤ Likes To Fight

1-10-12-2-15-17/18-22-14-24 ➤ Intermittent Argument

1-10-22-12-15-17/18-2-14-24 ➤ Lost Fight

9-22

When the bones and muscles (9) are in the same numerical chain as the parathyroid (22), it indicates that the person may be physically weak and is allowing his "unconfrontable" experiences to pile up. In other words, he is not accepting his experiences. He is letting them accrue on the physical body. When a person has an experience and it precipitates calcium, it must be removed from the physical body and translated into a mental aspect, translated into energies that are minute enough so as not to clash with physical substance.

Arthritics are individuals who refuse to accept experiences. They have unexpressed resentments. They are disgruntled about what has happened to them in the past, and they won't allow these experiences to be processed into their minds. Therefore, the calcium is kicked back out into the system and it knots up all the areas of the body that they won't accept. One of the most prominent areas with acceptance problems are the hands, and the area with the most rejection is the feet. So these two areas are hit first on the periphery by the kickback of calcium. It is essential for an individual who has a 9-22 in his chain to be sure that he processes his mind enough to accept the viewpoints of other people. If we were to look at the problem in store for someone with number 22, we would see that the transformation of anger into an experience that can be accepted by this person requires the ability to accept the viewpoint of the enemy: those who oppose him.

Physical Aspects

1-22

In an SAF chain, when the thymus (1) is present with the parathyroid (22), the individual may have bone troubles. His primary defenses have been breached and he is unable to coordinate and collect enough information on these occurrences into his mind so that they can reject the precipitation of calcium. If the individual is highly pressurized and a male dragon is chasing him, then his condition may develop into arthritis. On the other hand, if a female dragon is chasing him and that particular trauma takes energies (power) away from that person, then his bone troubles may be osteoporosis and cancer.

10-22

If the thyroid (10) is in the same SAF numerical chain as the parathyroid (22), the individual may be losing the capability for emotional experiences, and his spine may degenerate. The person may have low back troubles, pains in the low back, sciatica and other similar difficulties.

15-22

If the hypothalamus (15) and the parathyroid (22) are in the same SAF chain, the individual may be developing tumors. Poisons reach such a peak of concentration that pressure builds up in the experience tracts of the human being and begin to create a tornado-like energy, which is very advantageous to the creation of male and female dragons. The male dragon turns his tornado in clockwise, while the female dragon turns hers counterclockwise. The female and male dragons use this turning method to wrap energy up around themselves, in a ball-like fashion, to pull energy away from the body in the female sense, or push it in more closely in the male sense. When sick people say they have been "screwed," they are speaking the truth in an energy sense, because of the motion or pattern of attack. When the hypothalamus (15) is aligned with the parathyroid (22), it causes white body light or visible radiation to come into being. These miniature balls of energy become solid enough to make a tumor-like growth, especially on the bones and in the soft tissue surrounding the bones.

SAF Chains and 16-22 Combinations

22-16-1-5-10-12-13-17/18-14 ➤ gravel

1-10-12-13-17/18-14-16-22 ➤ old stones

16-1-5-10-12-13-17/18-14-22 ➤ new stone

1-5-10-12-22-16-17/18-14-13 ➤ gravel pain

22-1-5-10-16-17/18-14-13-12 ➤ dissolving stones

1-5-10-12-16-14-22-17/18-13 ➤ Stuck stones

1-22-10-5-14-16-17/18-13-12 ➤ diminishing stone

12-13-10-5-1-22-17/18-16-14 ➤ chronic gravel

16-22

Anytime the kidneys (16) are connected with the parathyroid (22), there are indications that this person is developing a process of solidification in the kidneys.

Kidney and bladder stones are formed from experiential energies that are part of this anger experience process. This individual refuses to allow the precipitates of calcium to be dissolved into his mind for acceptance.

It should always be noted that when 16-22, 15-22, or any number involving 22 is in the chain, the person is not in a mode to accept. He is constantly in the process of rejecting any other viewpoint but his own. When this occurs, the person has set himself up for a great liability because he is going into agreement with the dragon. Because the dragon is an experience all its own and has its own complete identity and personality, it won't accept any other reality.

The important thing is that if you can consistently change your viewpoint and your idea about circumstances, it will relieve pressure. A change of mind will allow energies to move into mental aspects. Solidification and tumors can't develop under these conditions. Tumor-like growths develop when a person refuses to see the other side, when he puts his attention on energies that he feels are justified to stay forever frozen in one position. This person's energies have been stuck in one particular picture and it is this effigy that causes a constant turning of energy to produce stones, tumors, growths and the like.

Because the dragon is an experience all its own and has its own complete identity and personality, it won't accept any other reality.

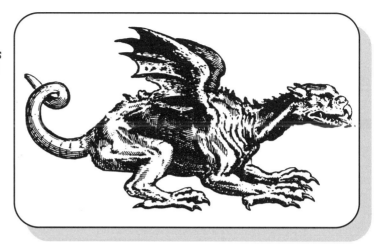

19-22

When the skin (19) and the parathyroid (22) cause a 19-22 sequence, the individual may be developing corns, calluses and hardened areas of the skin. These are produced when the individual refuses to let energies (chemicals, ideas) roam or circulate within the body. They move in a precise and complete circuit within themselves and develop their own entity as the offspring of dragons.

Does this mean that a person who has developed calluses and corns from playing sports or athletics has given room for the entrance of a dragon? Well, the idea is that the pressures brought to bear on the body have not been processed properly and those calluses build up for a reason. A person doesn't need any of those calluses. He may think he does because he is playing a sport and a callus protects his skin from blistering, but the skin is resilient and powerful enough to produce its own protective mechanism. It doesn't need to have an extra layer of hardened skin on it. Even so, an athletic callus could easily be a friendly, servicing dragon.

SAF Chains and (19)- (22) Combinations

4-6-10-<u>19</u>-<u>22</u>-12-14-15-20 ➤ hardened skin

2-<u>19</u>-<u>22</u>-4-6-10-12-14-15-20 ➤ callus

2-<u>22</u>-4-<u>19</u>-6-10-12-14-15-20 ➤ blister

<u>22</u>-2-10-12-14-<u>19</u>-15-20 ➤ mole

<u>19</u>-2-4-6-10-<u>22</u>-12-14-15-20 ➤ wart

4-6-10-<u>19</u>-12-14-15-20-<u>22</u> ➤ pimple

2-6-<u>22</u>-12-<u>19</u>-10-14-15-20 ➤ acne

<u>19</u>-2-4-6-10-12-14-15-<u>22</u> ➤ clear skin

23

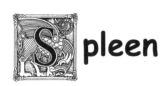pleen

The spleen is a gland-like organ that serves as a blood reservoir and is considered the garbage disposal for the tired blood cells, worn out erythrocytes, toxins and poisons. It sets hemoglobin free, produces lymphocytes and plasma cells, and also creates new erythrocytes for fetal life and newborns.

Emotion: Antagonism

When the number 23 appears in the numerical chain sequence created by the SAF techniques, the individual may exhibit signs and symptoms of chronic antagonism. He is the kind of individual who likes to tease and irritate other people. This is a petulant individual, but at the same time he doesn't have an extremely disastrous type of disease pattern. The higher numbers in the SAF programming, those from 20 to 24, are lighter in nature (disease patterns are less serious.) However, when an individual displays a 23, it certainly means that he could be having a hard time developing emotional patterns that are of a higher and more positive sort.

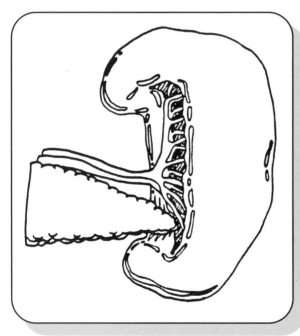

The Spleen

Condition: Rejection

People who show the acute inability to cope with the outside environment are primarily exhibiting patterns of allergies. When 23 appears in a numerical chain, it means that allergic conditions may exist, with a range of reactions from a skin rash to full blown anaphylactic shock, which is dangerous and/or deadly in certain circumstances. The breakdown of the immune system is the cause for the disturbances that abound around the number 23.

1-23

When the number 23 is found with the thymus (1) in a chain, the individual shows the highest danger of pressure, which may cause allergic reactions. Of course, the allergies may come from many different sources: food, the air, the water, contaminates, environmental pesticides, poisons, toxins, radiation, pollution and a plethora of energies in the environment that may provoke the allergic response reaction.

SAF Chains and 1-23 Combinations

1-23-24-2-10-3-9-15-22 ➤ allergies

24-2-10-3-1-23-9-15-22 ➤ worried about rejection

23-24-2-4-10-7-8-1-9 ➤ immunity

9-1-23-4-10-7-8-9-15-22 ➤ intermittent allergy

1-2-4-10-7-9-8-15-22-23 ➤ possible allergy

1-7-6-9-21-23-4-10-8-22 ➤ defense malfunction

2-23-4-10-20-5-1-8-9-22 ➤ relief (numbers reversed)

4-2-10-7-8-9-15-16-22-8-23-1 ➤ chronic remedy for allergy

In effect, the overabundance or pervasion of any substance in the environment can cause the allergic response. The body is rejecting poisons because it is aware that the energies (poisons and toxins) in the system for that particular wavelength and frequency have exceeded their normal amount. In the case of allergies, a signal is sent out in the form of dolor (pain), calor (heat), rubar (redness), and tumor (swelling).

In a sense, this immune system is on full amplification. It is better for a human being to have an allergic reaction than to permit the insidious entrance of toxins without any reaction at all. In effect, the allergic response is the exhibition of black body mass and black body radiation, which alerts the rest of the immune system.

When dragons enter through black body mass and black body radiation, the individual may not realize he has been invaded, a situation that can be much more detrimental than an allergy. However, people are uncomfortable and complain that their symptoms are more highly amplified than when they observe the allergy signal.

The reason a person has an allergy in the first place is because he has not paid enough attention to the earlier signs and symptoms presented to him by his immune system. Symptoms are sending a message. He has probably used drugs to cover his symptoms, hiding his troubles with creams, aspirin and all manner of medicinal drug devices and appliances to prevent his body from signaling him with the proper information as to the type of poison that entered his system. But even so, allergic individuals are luckier than are others who have severe illnesses because they still maintain the ability to reject toxins and poisons.

7-23

When the lungs (7) are connected with the spleen (23), the person may display signs of asthma, lung allergies and bronchitis. Different poisons involving the breathing apparatus can be found when observing the 7-23 combinations in a chain.

Mental Aspects

When 23 appears in a SAF chain, the person may exhibit the mental attitude or atmosphere of rejection. He may have rejected someone, or someone else may have rejected him. He could have been in the vicinity of a rejection of someone he loved, such as the type of rejection that occurs between brother and sister, or mother and father, or someone else close to him. Rejection is a powerful action. Many cases, however, are caused by problems of <u>detoxification</u>, the colon (3). In this case, the person's inability to reject toxins and poisons causes the buildup of the emotional state of hatred. We find that his colon (3) problem can often be solved with help from the spleen (23). The individual can thoroughly reject toxins, poisons and those things that he believes to be detrimental to himself.

2-23

Where the whole mechanism goes haywire is when the person rejects the wrong target, or is rejected for the wrong reason, or when the action of rejection is a puzzlement. In this case, we obtain a twisted view of life because it is generally believed that "bad" is to be rejected and "good" accepted. Many times in the environment, we can behave the best that we can behave (be good) and still experience rejection. This is true when the heart (2) is in the same chain as the spleen (23). In a sense, the person has had a rejection and the whole sequence of numbers oriented to the heart (2) will give us the exact diagram or blueprint of separations, losses, divorces and disturbances in the environment that break people apart and cause traumatic experiences (female dragons). The rejection of love (2-23) is a very easy action to experience because people misconstrue love behavior on a daily basis. Rejection is something that occurs quite easily and with rejection comes anger at the loved one (2-22). Finally, a total loss or separation of the person is allowed and leaves an imprint on that person's consciousness. This is called the loss of a loved one, (2-20).

We can easily reject ideas, programs, plans and even our own purpose or goals - mistakenly. It is the project of SAF to re-acquaint individuals to their purposes and their plans for life. If we go astray from the primary directives for our existence, we are liable to create havoc with our present condition.

Physical Aspects

The individual with a 23 in the front of the chain may exhibit breathing difficulties, rashes, pimples, swelling, redness and have pains in the joints. You might not realize that allergies can cause arthritis and rheumatoid situations. The allergies may come from eating foods, drinking certain water or water in general, or breathing the air. As was described in the previous paragraph, there may be cerebral and mental allergies occurring from rejection states and other stress patterns with which you can't cope.

7-23

When the lungs (7) are associated with the spleen (23) in the same numerical chain, there is a possibility that the individual will develop an asthmatic condition, breathing difficulties or troubles that may lead to a chronic bronchial situation. The wrong thing to do is to spend time and money on drug programs for this merely suppresses the toxins and the poisons of the drugs earlier ingested, which are the real cause of the trouble. Individuals who have taken too much adrenaline for asthmatic conditions find that their tissues become wasted of water and the skin displays coppery spots as a result of poisons that have nestled in the colon (3).

23-24

When the spleen (23) is connected with the lymph (24), then we observe a genetic changeover. This means that whatever conditions (numbers) lie between these two numbers in a numerical chain, these symptoms, signs and signals are part of a genetic hand-me-down or a hereditary "legacy."

A legacy is something that we are given by our ancestors to solve while living with our present human body. Although most don't realize it, many of the conditions we try to solve are age-old conditions that our genetic line developed as long ago as 500,000 years. Each gene assigns each generation a riddle to solve. It is well nigh impossible for an ordinary human being to come up with remedies for these particular genetic problems.

Adding contemporary drugs and medicines to this factor will defeat the person trying to solve his problems. We can only try to hedge against whatever the genetic troubles seem to be. For example, we may have asthma, breathing difficulties, diabetes, alcoholism, syphilis and gonorrhea, bone troubles, chronic headaches and the like. This is just a small list of what could be handed down from one generation to the next.

Because the genetic code has collected all the historical ancestral memory banks, which have come in contact with physical bodies, minds and the memory deposits of all experienced life, then almost anything can be handed down. It seems that these genetic propensities will carry through if they have a greater concentration than other diseases or maladies in the system. This is a scientific fact. It is not guess work. An alcoholic mother will give birth to an alcoholic child.

It is up to the individual in his lifetime to try to control these impulses, but it can be very difficult. If he doesn't have SAF programming and the techniques delivered by the Self Awareness Formulas, then he certainly won't figure out the codes he needs to break this alcoholic pattern. All he could do is stay away from alcohol. The real miracle would be to edit the problem out of the genetic sense-mechanisms of the body and have the person be able to socialize again without becoming a roaring drunkard. It is proposed that with SAF, this is possible.

> *Once a SAFent has become aware of the dragon's existence, his own energies become irradiated with mental awareness fires powerful enough to dematerialize a dragon and all his symptoms. The SAFent acquires new tranquility in his resting places.*

24

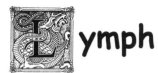ymph

Lymph, composed of lymphocytes, is a transparent, slightly yellow liquid found in lymphatic vessels throughout the body. Its purpose is to cleanse the body of toxins, especially those in the blood system. Because the body is made up of almost 85% fluid, it is essential that there be a mechanism in place to process systemic toxins and poisons. Lymph nodes or relay centers hold and process poisons then release them through the skin and sweat glands.

Emotion: Enthusiasm

The number 24 often appears in a chain when individuals exhibit exhilaration or an excitement to do any kind of program. Whatever number 24 appears next to in a chain gives us a clue as to the program. We find that the person is interested in applying some remedy or outside mechanism other than the willpower of his mind.

We see that 24 is used primarily with concentrations and also dependencies of certain drug materials. However, what is considered a drug in SAF programs is any material or method used outside the willpower of the individual. This means cigarettes, coffee, tea and even vitamins could be blamed. Many of the drug substances that have been detected have been materials such as marijuana, LSD, cocaine, crack, smack, heroin, mescaline and all prescription drugs. Sometimes a person gets confused when asked if he is taking drugs. We automatically think "drugs" is a term used for street drugs or controlled substances.

In reality, drugs can be any kind of outside material or

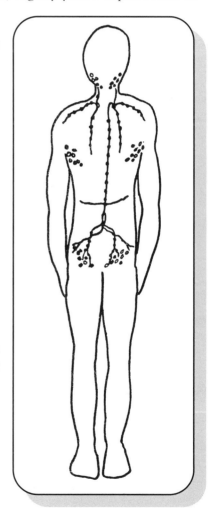

The Lymph System

method exerting control on the human system. Exercise, done excessively, can act as a drug. So can meditation or yoga. In fact, meditation is one of the stronger drugs that is employed because it affects the mind and therefore directs the energies of the body to perform. Yoga is a form of meditation. So we must be mindful of those who are exercising or meditating obsessively. When 24 appears in a chain, it means that some kind of action is being used against a situation, whatever it is.

6-24

In most cases, the 24 appears right next to the numbers of the troubled organs that the person is trying to treat. For example, if a person is taking a liver medicine, then the number 6 (liver) will appear right before the number 24 (lymph) to indicate that the person is taking a drug or remedy and it is affecting the liver.

3-24

Sometimes coffee reacts in this way and appears next to the colon (3) in the SAF chain, reading as 3-24.

Condition: Acceptance

The opposite of rejection is acceptance. It means the individual is willing to accept any program that is brought before him. Often when the number 24 appears in the chain it indicates that the individual has over-accepted many programs, and these program toxins and materials have actually gone too far; they are affecting the system overtly without the person's awareness.

Many times people attuned to a healthy lifestyle are taken aback when the SAF Monitor asks them if they have been taking some kind of drug. They respond with "No! I never take drugs." At the same time they are piling vitamins in left and right. They believe that these vitamins are not acting like a drug.

Drug, in SAF terminology, is the past tense of "drag." It means the person is putting some drag on his problem. In other words, he feels his symptoms are racing ahead of him too fast. He can't take the pain, the pressure or the sensation. He doesn't like the way he feels, so he puts a little drag on the condition. Drag is something needed and wanted by the person to slow down the electrical charges of the condition.

The SAF definition of drag can be found in physics and in the science of electrical engineering where a technician uses a resistor to put drag on an electrical circuit. It is called "doping" the circuit to slow it down. The technician doesn't want to put high-powered electrical energy into machines that may overload so he needs resistors or other kinds of electrical equipment to "dope" a circuit and slow down the electrical input.

This is the same action that a human being wants to accomplish - to slow down the electrical energy that has entered his body. He may remember an event in his life that contained a little too much electricity for him to handle. He may feel "scorched" when he thinks of his ex- wife, for example. He may have a big speech to give in front of a large audience, or he may have had some catastrophe or disaster befall him. These mental images of the events carry too much electrical charge and can overload his circuits, so he resorts to drugs to "dope" his circuits. He slows down the electrical charges so he can cope with them. This doesn't seem like a wrong thing to do, but if we overload our system in such a way, when we do want to have a high powered electrical circuit, it won't be there. We will have too much poison and toxin in the system.

There are other books that discuss chemicals and substances that affect the humanoid system. Homeopathic drugs can be used because they are diluted enough to do one or two "dopings" and then leave. When an individual imbibes concentrated drugs and materials, the consolidation effect causes a condition that results in thousands of dopings per dosage. This means that the doping effect will last much longer than is necessary. Some people take so many drugs and medicines into their systems to create a doping effect that they have enough dosages there to last a thousand years, long after the body is dead.

Mental Aspects

The individual who exhibits a number 24 in his chain is exuberant, happy and alive. He is excited and exhilarated. The word enthusiasm is used because any kind of remedy that is found, and works to any degree, is exactly what a person likes. This is why alcohol can be such an exuberant remedy. No one uses a droll, resigned tone when they say, "Let's go get drunk." A person who appreciates the medicinal effect of liquor exclaims, "Let's get bombed!!" and then shouts "whoopee!" At the end of a long day of punching cows out in the New Mexico desert, the cowboys race back home for a nice cold beer.

Whatever the remedy, number 24 individuals are constantly enthusiastic about it; they race for it, even something as simple to quench as thirst. If the individual is thirsty enough, he will certainly become enthusiastic about drinking water. If a person has a headache, he is quite enthusiastic about reaching the right remedy. As the head pain pulses harder and harder, he will do just about anything to get rid of it. If we were to suggest that a certain little pill was capable of getting rid of the headache, he would certainly take it enthusiastically, no matter what the consequences.

This, of course, is the mind-set of most individuals existing on the planet Earth today. For the most part, people have not given any consideration to the ramifications of what would happen to their bodies and their energies (genetic) down the line. They are mainly enthusiastic for handling or remedying situations in the present, no matter what chemical substances are needed.

However, we should be much more diligent about what we put into our body. By understanding exactly how the body functions, we can take the right dosage of remedy. We can use the right "doping plan" to slow down energies in certain circumstances and then let go of this doping so that we can again gain power.

Some of today's citizens are completely benumbed, falling apart, exhausted and lacking any energy or drive because they overdosed themselves 10, 15 or 20 years ago. People who are consistently doping themselves do so because their energies (mind and body) are keyed in to their present drug use. They run on mechanical advice and are acting like zombies, for their energy is dependent upon the drugs they are taking. Many have trapped themselves into taking one pill to calm down and another to excite them. They have certainly fallen victim to the over-doping, overdosing merry-go-round.

Physical Aspects

2-24

When the heart (2) is aligned with the lymph (24) a person may have breathing difficulties or cardiac troubles. When overdoses of toxic materials (drugs) get into his system, it directly affects the synchronization of his body.

If the person overdoses his drugs, he is in chronic danger of re-experiencing those same toxins. Any single dose of medication on the market today – one pill, one tablespoon of medicine – is an overdose of possibly a thousand times more than we actually need. This fact has been proven for over two hundred years, by perhaps millions of people. A glance at the "drug insert" literature for prescription drugs, or the label of over-the-counter medicines will tell us just how potent these products are.

Take, for example, a person who smoked marijuana in college. The tars, resins and the overdose of the concentrated smoke that were drawn into his lungs at that time can re-ignite and cause the person the same feelings (symptoms) when he least expects it. A person at forty-five years of age, who hasn't smoked marijuana in 20 years, could suddenly exhibit all the symptoms of being "stoned." Only it was so long ago, he doesn't realize what it is. He thinks he's crazy. This is not uncommon. People who formerly took stronger, more concentrated drugs such as LSD are even more likely to have an attack (a trip) again without suspecting the cause.

15-24

Many people who took drugs in the past have one foot in reality and one foot in hallucination. They have a chronic sense perception problem. When the hypothalamus (15) is near the lymph (24) on a chain, we know that the person has had drug experiences that have affected his senses. His sense perceptions are askew.

5-24

If the anterior pituitary (5) is in the SAF chain, then it is known that the drugs are affecting the person's control of reality. He may look at a fish and see an apple. He may look at a banana and see a boat. He may hear certain words uttered (by a family member or business associate) and receive the sounds as a completely different thought.

These people can't be trusted in any circumstance. They are liable to make one big error in their lives. This is always the case when we try to fathom why a person of reasonable intelligence becomes a victim of some bizarre accident or strange coincidence of events or traumas.

If LSD gets into someone's system and disturbs the micro-fine mechanisms that control the chromosomes of that body, then not only does it affect the past and the present of that human being, but also his future. We can inadvertently program into our genes our own demise in a fantastic and horrible way.

Individuals who have spent time experimenting with drugs don't realize the intense powder keg of energy that they have created. It is necessary for them to spend time understanding, dissecting, solving and sorting out the riddles of these drugs so that they can remove the erroneous programming that has entered their systems. If we can pull the plug on the drugs that are already in the system, then we have a fighting chance at being able to live in some sense of reality. As long as the drugs are inside a person's body, they can work their energies into the system and actually reprogram the human being for disaster. If a SAFent wonders why he or she had or is having bad luck, it may all be coming from a preset program developed by the inner connection and the chemical bonding of drugs that entered the body long ago. It could be from the drugs given to the mother at his or her birth or from seventy-five years previous as in a genetic hand-me-down.

23-24

When the spleen (23) is connected to the lymph (24), the drug situation is worse than anyone had ever thought possible. The person has actually inherited the hand-me-down drug problem. This is, of course, entirely true in the case of alcoholics. It is wholly possible that even drugs such as penicillin and antibiotics can be handed down. For example, if a person has an allergy to penicillin and has offspring, those descendants may also have the allergy to penicillin.

For the record, the author is thoroughly convinced that any trait, quirk or disorder that your mother or father had, the offspring acquires as well. It is a matter of the concentration of the particular problem. In each individual life these traits, disorders and toxins take on a specific order of priority. You may not have the same order of priority of dissecting a particular problem that your ancestors had, and we never know how far back on the family tree cancer, tumors, arthritis, diabetes or whatever the trauma dragon, first surfaced. Some of these conditions may be on a 200-year cycle so that none of the immediate ancestors (mother, grandfather, etc.) are known to have had the disorder.

Genetic research is just now coming in vogue, so it will be several generations before enough statistical data can be codified to authenticate exactly what diseases, viruses, drugs, X-rays, etc. will have adverse effects on future generations.

Although the "common man" is only beginning to be examined by such genetic counselors, the royal families of Europe, interested in keeping blood lines blue (royal), have amassed much data on genetics. In addition to scanty physician records, certain personality disorders of prominent kings and queens were written down for posterity, and these biographies have become another method used by modern investigators to trace family diseases and imbalances.

Two hereditary diseases were found through modern day methods and traced back by descriptions of personalities to 1542 AD. The end result showed afflicted kings, queens, dukes, princes and emperors of England, Prussia, Germany, Spain and Russia.

One disease, porphyria, is a metabolic condition evidenced by gastrointestinal dysfunction, neurological disturbances, and the passing of red urine as the blood cells lose their rosy hue. These royal personages did indeed have less red-colored blood – and presumably more blue – than their countrymen did.

A second disease traced was hemophilia, which affected princes in Prussia, Spain, England and Russia. Queen Victoria, a direct descendant of porphyria victims and carriers, passed hemophilia on to her progeny. Hemophilia is a blood disorder where the clotting factor VIII is low resulting in hemorrhaging. Scientists have speculated that a mutant gene was responsible for this disorder, as previous instances of "bleeders" were not known in Victoria's family.

Could this hemophilia gene have been mutated by the DNA/RNA as a result of weakened cell structure caused by previous generations afflicted with porphyria? What of the attitudes and emotions that predispose us to certain disorders and ailments? Are these also inheritable?

Does each generation pass on to their progeny a drug-dependence syndrome, alcoholism, X-ray build-up, or physical and mental reactions to stimuli?

It is the author's contention that this is precisely what occurs. All emotions, attitudes and personality quirks are just as easily transmitted to future generations as are physical disorders and characteristics, via the genetic blueprint as contained in the DNA/RNA. It is also postulated that these instances, anomalies and disorders can be found and uncovered with SAF programming, opening further the doors to eugenics.

"The numerical matrix of the sun can be used in a proven mathematical formula to help you gain insight into your troubles."

— Joseph R. Scogna, Jr.

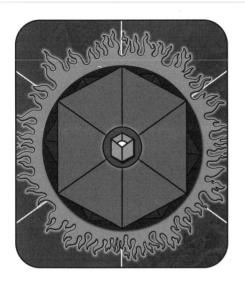

Chapter 6

How to Read the SAF Chain

In This Chapter

➤ Chain reaction of energy
➤ Chain logic – lead, core, anchor
➤ Present time versus the past
➤ Every chain has a story
➤ How to read the chain, or pulling the dragon's tail
➤ SAF Simplified worksheet
➤ Tamper/SAF Operative Chart
➤ SAF Stress – 120 Questionnaire

The numerical chain has been given a great deal of mention thus far. At this point, the specifics of its creation and operation will be explained.

The SAF chain is a particular sequence of numbers read from the left to the right and from the right to the left. The greatest <u>effect</u> can be found on the left and the greatest <u>cause</u> is depicted on the right side of the chain.

Chain Reaction of Energy

As was previously discussed, the exact energy sequence from the sun, throughout the spaces around the sun, including the planet Earth, creates a specific chain reaction of energy that affects the organ and gland systems of a human being in a precise order. That order is as follows:

1. Thymus
2. Heart
3. Colon
4. Stomach
5. Anterior Pituitary
6. Liver
7. Lungs
8. Sex Organs
9. Bones and Muscles
10. Thyroid & Veins and Arteries of the Upper Extremities
11. Veins & Arteries of the Lower Extremities
12. Brain
13. Adrenal Glands
14. Mind
15. Hypothalamus and the Senses
16. Kidneys
17/18. Endocrine System
19. Skin
20. Pancreas & Solar Plexus
21. Posterior Pituitary
22. Parathyroid
23. Spleen
24. Lymph System

This rundown is a sequence or a chain itself. Each individual organ is linked to the next, similar to a chain of iron links.

The Sun and Its Significance

The energies of humankind and the energies of physical environmental natures around human beings co-exist in partnership. We create our own world while the sun and stars create the specific magnetic blueprint of the physical universe. Somewhere in between the two creations lies the co-existence and the harmony. As energies are moved from one system to the next in a complete harmonizing focus following the sun's blueprint, the energies of the genetic blueprint of each of us, as well as our mind and spirit, dreams, wishes, whims and intentions are programmed against the energies of the sun.

When a numerical chain is constructed by SAF techniques, it should not be in sequential order, such as 2-3-4-5-6-7. Any piece of the sun's sequence (1-2-3-4-5-6-7) or (7-8-9-10-11-12-13) belongs to the <u>sun</u> and not a human being. Human chains or numbers should be scrambled, such as 5-12-9-3-24-21-11. If our chain mimics the sun or goes into phase with the energy of the sun, this means that the sun is reclaiming our energies.

In all cases where a SAFent showed a numerical chain in the exact sequence of the sun's energy, he was already listed as a psychotic. In effect, there was no mind there; there was no spirit guiding the body. When the body is completely in a zombie-like condition, the numbers will read in a chain sequence such as 1-2-3-4-5, or 10-11-12-13-14-15, or 21-22-23-24.

When there is some entity – a spirit, a will or a desire overcoming the body's energies – then the numbers will be mixed, they will be erratic, showing that organs are over-heating in different patterns. Then the SAF Monitor will have something with which to work.

Earth Patterns: Disease Patterns

In SAF, a chain is written as a universal arithmetical expression. Because numbers have absolutely no personality in themselves, and because numbers are merely a pressure gradation from 1 to infinity, we need to assign some importance to these number factors to cause them to be useful.

The SAF project has developed a vast information bank on the various patterns and sequences of numbers created against the organ systems by the interaction and interposition of certain entities in the environment, such as foods, minerals, air, water, etc. This project has already catalogued several million sequences to allow a SAFent to track or follow any effect that a dragon (trauma) may have upon the human body.

For example, the diabetes dragon has a code number: 1-6-13-17/18-21. The arthritis dragon has a code number 1-9-22. An apple also has a code number: 5-11-13-21. A car has a code number and so do a bird and a dog. In short, any object, animal, vegetable, mineral, or artificially created material has a code number.

Dragon Types

The code numbers are developed when they are interconnected with the human system, and the trauma or dragon energies (people, places and things) have a tendency to heat up certain organs. The whole purpose of the sun's radiant chain, that is, the numbers that affect the organs in their proper sequence, such as thymus, heart, colon, stomach, etc., is a gradation of hot to cold.

When a trauma-dragon intersects with the body, how many organs and glands will be heated up? How many organs are significant? By the massive research that was compiled on the SAF project, the specific sequence of energy has been set forth to allow a person to realize the exact extent of radiational exposure to a human body. There can be one or two organs affected, as is most often depicted in this book. Tri-numeric expressions (three numbers) are more complex followed by quadra-numeric and then penta-numeric. According to SAF principles, the highest expression of trauma that can exist is a six number expression. This means there will be six organs and glands affected in sequence.

Each SAF chain possesses a story about the effect of traumas on the human being; it is a self awareness tool.

The problem is in trying to translate what kind of dragon is intersecting with the body.

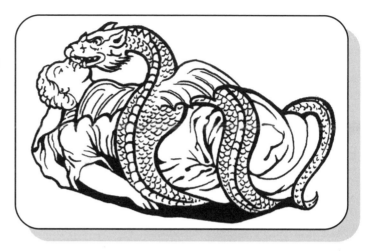

For example, when an SAF chain is produced with a number (4) logged as the first number, it indicates that (4), the stomach, is the hottest area on the chain. Remember that two entities can't occupy the same space at the same time, so when two entities, such as the stomach and some paranormal toxin infesting the stomach tissues, try to occupy the same space at the same time, a predictable reaction occurs- heat is produced.

As described earlier in this text, whenever an entity or energy gets lodged in the body, it will produce dolor (pain), calor (heat), rubar (redness), and tumor (swelling). It really doesn't matter whether the rubar or the tumor is existent, but it does matter if there is pain or heat present because this differentiates whether the dragon is male or female. If you have heat or pressure in that location, then there is a male dragon. If you have a spot of coldness, there is a female dragon, one which is drawing energy (cells, tissue, molecules) away from the body.

The whole trick of the SAF program is to effectively translate the information in the SAF numeric chain sequence from an <u>arithmetical expression</u> into a <u>grammatical expression</u>. For this reason, the manner in which the chain is constructed causes a breakthrough in language between non-speaking entities.

The biggest breakthrough for the deaf to be able to communicate was sign language, and for the blind it was the development of the Braille system. Each system enabled those afflicted to communicate where previously silence had reigned supreme.

The SAF system is a similar breakthrough because it gives people the ability to speak and communicate with disease entities and past traumas. Its basic principle of operation is a system of hot and cold, but the chain links have specific rules and regulations that cause the existence of a particular sequence of words that must be grammatically correct to enable the SAFent and SAF Monitor total understanding.

The Chain, or Finding the Dragon's Tail

There can be twelve numbers in a chain. If the chain is shorter than twelve numbers, it indicates that the recording tracks are smothered and you may be in a state of over-whelm. In this case, several tracks may be squashed together and read as one, or they may be dissected and cut off from your reality.

In subjective questioning using the Stress-120 Questionnaire, you may have a single number in a chain, but this is a dis-reality coming from your imagination.

If you have more than twelve numbers in a chain, such as 14, 15 or 16 numbers, it indicates that you are picking up recording tracks. You are borrowing energy from another entity and using it as your own.

Technicians in the science of healing, including doctors, massage therapists, acupunc-turists, chiropractors, reflexologists, and those who spend their time touching other people, will often have more than the twelve numbers in a chain because they are picking up "phantom recording tracks." These phantom recording tracks come from the frictional energy that produces a mirror image of the recording track. A practitioner of the healing arts, by touching, "copied" an experience of the person they touched. In such a chain, the SAF practitioner is seeing a ghost. However, when running such a program, we must pay attention to these ghosts because they do have some connec-tion to the SAFent and must be acknowledged.

A simple chain of numbers can produce an almost incredible amount of information. The numbers move across 880 subject banks, which means that each number from 1 to 24 (thymus to lymph) can have 880 various meanings depending upon which subject bank is chosen. Some of these are: color, sound, food, energy, vitamins, minerals, enzymes, glandular preparations, emotions, fears, conditions, situations, business, etc. The list goes on and on, covering 880 subjects known to mankind. In this book, the reading of your chain will be more simplistic but other books are available for those interested in further study.

Chain Logic
Lead – Core – Anchor

In a chain, the first number on the left is the lead number, and the last number on the right is the anchor number. The very center number (in a chain with an odd amount of numbers) or center two numbers (in an even number chain) is the core. Comprehen-sion of the lead, core and anchor is necessary for understanding the SAF program.

Odd Number Chain:
<u>10</u> - 9 - 1 - 2 - **<u>4</u>** - 16 - 12 - 13 - **<u>17/18</u>**
lead   core   anchor

Even Number Chain:
<u>17/18</u> - 20 - 14 - 15 - **<u>16 - 1</u>** - 3 - 6 - 9 - **<u>10</u>**
lead   core #s   anchor

Present Time versus In the Past

The major differentiation between the two halves of the chain is that the left side is the hottest, occurring right now, while the right side is the coolest, and happened in the past.

The Chain is a Trauma Entity

In understanding the SAF chain we understand life. The chain is actually presenting a "slice of life" to examine and understand. Students of SAF have always been cautioned to be careful when working with these chains because they are alive and viable for the SAFent. The specific sequence of organ degeneration from 1 to 24 ignites a particular pattern so that seeing numbers in these chains stimulates a certain hailing frequency for trauma dragons. In other words, a person can call his own unconscious traumas forward with these sequences of numbers. For this reason, it is important to remember that while studying chains it is best to remain detached from the chains of other people.

Another word of caution: do not try to obtain several chains on yourself at once. Work on the first chain until you understand it and have gained more awareness about yourself and the SAF program.

The chain itself is a dragon entity.

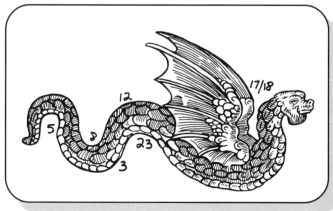

Start to Finish

When you decide to fill out a questionnaire and run a chain (attack the dragon, so to speak) do so with a definite intention to start the chain and a definite intention to end it. These chains should never be run if you do not intend to fully complete what you start. If you start the chain and don't finish it, over time it may build extra electric/magnetic momentum, creating enough energy for the dragon to put down roots. In other words, traumas will be stimulated. When this occurs, they are in the visible light spectrum and reside in the present reality. In essence, you will be re-living your trauma. The ideal scenario is for you to locate this trauma and identify its parts, which releases the electromagnetic charge. Once the charge is released, you will gain new understandings and feel relief.

So again, caution is advised.

➤ Study these chains in a detached manner

➤ Take one chain at a time

➤ Finish what you start

Every Chain Has A Story

The chain and its factors have been fashioned after the grammatical sciences learned in elementary school through the college level. In this book we will pay attention to the lead, the core and the anchor numbers, as well as a few of the up-links listed in chapter 5.

Remember sentence structure from your school days? Based on English language usage and thought processes, sentences contain a subject, an object and a verb. And so it is with the SAF chain structure. The subject of the chain is the core number, the lead number is the object, and the anchor number is the verb of the chain sentence.

The string of numbers is translated and read as a grammatical sentence. In effect, in every chain there is a story, a story about the SAFent. Some stories are extremely long – novel length – while others are short stories or just a few words long. It depends on the expertise of the SAF Monitor in writing the story, the chain biography, for the SAFent. But please note, if you follow this book it is not necessary to work under an SAF Monitor.

If this is your first experience with SAF, you will most likely want to "talk to" that particular upset that is plaguing your body – we call this your major complaint. Because these trauma dragons can't be destroyed by drugs (even though many scientists think this is what occurs), we must work out some arrangement to find out what the entity (trauma) is attempting to tell you. Remember that there is no such thing as bad energy, there is only energy from experiences and events that gets confused and mixed up. With the mechanisms and technology of SAF, we can de-confuse energy.

Why Get a Major Complaint?

Stating a major complaint is mandatory or the chain biography is all for naught. We can just shoot in the dark and say this or that is the SAFent's problem, but we must always have a major complaint for reference.

A SAFent has to come forward and say, "I have a headache" or "I've got some problem with my digestive system." The trouble must be logged in first. If the bits of information from the chain biography don't relate to a SAFent's problem the chain won't make sense. And besides, if "nothing is wrong" then why spend the time trying to fix or understand "nothing"?

In the final analysis, it is important because we are trying to teach a SAFent (you) something about your dragon-trauma. We are trying to find the key that will unlock the mysteries of confusion. The challenge is there but YOU are the main ingredient. The major complaint can include emotions, the environment, attitudes, symptoms, problems, upsets, disease, or a present day distress of any kind.

Now you are ready to begin your own self awareness work. With that major complaint in mind, you will begin work on the SAF Simplified Worksheet and follow those directions.

"SAFents who have brought many dragons into the light are magnificent."

SAF Simplified Worksheet

Right now you must think about that situation or that confusion of energy that is getting in your way, your major complaint.

1._____Write: My present day major complaint is _____.

2._____Do: Insert the CD-ROM into your computer (IBM or MAC). It will start automatically.

3._____Read: the Copyright notice on the screen.

4._____Click: the START button.

5._____Answer: the SAF Stress – 120 Questionnaire on your screen.

When you click the FINISH button, your SAF chain will appear on the screen, as well as your lead, core and anchor numbers.

6._____Write: Your SAF chain:_____

List: your lead number:_____

List your core number(s): _____

List your anchor number: _____

7._____Use: the Tamper/SAF Operative Chart (page 211) to find the correct words.

List your lead word (condition)_____

List your core organ or gland _____

List your anchor word (emotion) _____

8._____Read: How to Read the Chain, or Pulling the Dragon's Tail, page 206-208.

The core is addressed first.

9._____Read: The complete section in Chapter 5 that relates to your core number(s).

10.____Ask: How does (_____) relate to/cause _____?
               Core organ word/explanation   present day complaint

If there are two numbers in the core, take the left number first, then the right number. Find a recent incident when this occurred.

Lead number is addressed second.

11. ____Read: the section in Chapter 5 that relates to the condition of your lead number.

12. ____Ask: How does (_____) relate to/cause _____?
                              Lead condition word   present day complaint

Anchor number is worked on last.

13. ____Read the section in Chapter 5 that relates to the emotion of your anchor number.

14. ____Ask: How does _____ relate to/cause _____?
                              Anchor emotion word   core and present day complaint

Once you have a recent time this occurred, you might be surprised to suddenly remember there was an earlier time these same emotions occurred also.

15. ____Read: Significant Up-Links, page 208.

16. ____Locate: any up-links in your chain.

Up-link _____ Description: _____ Up-link: _____ Description: _____

Up-link _____ Description: _____ Up-link: _____ Description: _____

Congratulations! You've just learned the rudiments on how to make and read an SAF chain. If there are any problems go back and make sure you finished each step in order. Read the case study on page 208.

Once you understand the steps of making a grammatical sentence out of the SAF numbers, the process gets easier. Once you start making cause and effect connections between your mental, physical and spiritual state, your energy will increase.

Now, write down what you have learned about yourself, your major complaint and the connections you have made.

_____

_____

_____

You can stop here, or continue with another chain. Make sure you use a different major complaint.

NOTE: this work sheet may be copied for additional SAF chain work.

How to read the Chain, or Pulling the Dragon's Tail

All chains are made into grammatical sentences based on English language usage.

➤ Core number is considered the subject

➤ Lead number is considered the object

➤ Anchor number is considered the verb

➤ The numbers in between the lead, the core and the anchor are called transients (for more definitive programming)

➤ The left side (lead number) indicates the present time

➤ The right side (anchor number) indicates the deep past, the first time this particular problem occurred.

➤ The core indicates a timeless state, not affected by time whatsoever. A core can't be past, present, or even future; it is "always" and "never" at the same time.

➤ By studying the Tamper/SAF Operative Chart we can range back and forth from the organ to the emotion to the condition and will be quite able to read chains on an elementary level.

➤ Significant up-links indicate syndromes or sequences of energy

The Core Number is the Subject

When reading a chain sentence, the core number is the subject of the sentence, what this chain is all about. You may not be fully aware that you have your mind on the core situation because the chain is viewing the dragon or trauma state, not your state. However, about five times out of six, the SAFent will know he has the core condition and is amazed that the program is able to make these connections for him.

FOR YOUR OWN CHAIN: From the Tamper/SAF Operative Chart (pg. 211), find the organ or gland word that fits your number. Write this down on the worksheet.

Reread the complete section in Chapter 5 that explains your core number (for example, if "10" then read chapter 5-10. This is the subject of your chain. Fill in the worksheet where requested.

The Lead Number is the Object (Effect)

When reading a chain sentence, the lead is the present reality, the result, or the effect. The lead number tells us what things are coming into being, what things are in the visible light spectrum and you will be more aware of them.

The lead number should be or match your major complaint, the symptom or the present day distress. It should be very visible and should be felt by you. The lead number indicates that this symptom should be the hottest and have the most pressure. If we follow the precepts of the forefathers of medicine, if enough calor (heat) is present then a good deal of dolar (pain), rubar (redness) and tumor (swelling) will be evident. The more heat buildup on that particular system, the more the energy will expose itself and will cause you to have discomfort. This discomfort and dis-ease will cause you to complain, and so this should be your major complaint.

If you do not recognize the connection, this is an indication that your energies (perceptions) are deeply buried.

FOR YOUR OWN CHAIN: From the Tamper/SAF Operative Chart (pg. 211), find the condition listed for your lead number. Write this down on the worksheet.

Re-read the condition section in chapter 5 that explains your lead number. Fill in the worksheet where requested.

The Anchor Number is the Verb

When reading the chain sentence, the anchor is the verb, the action word, the how and why something was done. It is the item that exposes the invisible energies, which allow the subject (core) to create the object (lead). So the anchor could be considered the ultimate physical cause.

This anchor number holds the pieces of this trauma in place. It gives the trauma its power over you. It is also the most occluded, the most hidden, but with the SAF Operative words and following the sentence structure, you can uncover its mysteries and release the electromagnetic charge from this chain.

FOR YOUR OWN CHAIN: From the Tamper/SAF Operative Chart (pg. 211), find the emotion listed for your anchor number. Write this down on the worksheet.

Re-read the emotion section in chapter 5 that explains your anchor number. Fill in the worksheet where requested.

Dual Cause

For further chain work, note there is a dual causal action focused on the object (lead number). There is the causal action of the subject and the causal action of the verb.

For example, in a scenario of building a house, the finished house is the object (lead) and the verb (anchor) is the action of the tools – the hammer strokes and nails. The subject (core) would be the carpenter wanting to create a house. So would we say that the hammer and nails built the house or the carpenter built the house? The carpenter did, but the hammer and nails were used. All three aspects are essential and work together for the finished product.

We look to the anchor number constantly to see how it was done, because by short circuiting these casual actions on the right (anchor), a smart SAF Monitor or SAFent will take most of the energy (cause) away from a dragon by taking his tools from him. If the fire is taken away from the dragon, he doesn't have nearly as much sting.

NOTE: If the lead and core words are addressed ONLY, the present day complaint charges up (+), and bothers the SAFent more. By successfully handling the anchor emotion, the dragon is charged up (+), enabling the SAFent to see it. After that the present day complaint discharges (-). The anchor emotion can be seen after working the core and lead words first.

Significant up-links

Finding the up-links in your chain will give you additional information. An up-link is two or more numbers in succession that ascend in value, such as 2-10, 4-16, and 14-15-17/18. These are listed throughout the book (check the index). These up-links indicate syndromes, or particular sequences of energy that will shed more light on your chain.

2-10 = break up, separation, or loss

4-16 = digestion is off

14-15-17/18 = business troubles

SAF Case Study

Major complaint: "problems with job"

5-4-6-<u>10</u>-12-14-<u>22</u>

Core: We look at the 10 first, the subject of this chain. The number 10 indicates the thyroid gland. Chapter 5-10 on thyroid explains that a SAFent with this chain has his attention on things that are changing and he's anxious about change.

Q. How could being <u>anxious about change</u> cause me to have <u>problems with job</u>?

Lead: For the lead number (5) we find the condition listed on the Tamper/SAF Operative Chart, which is coordination, the ability of the SAFent to keep things under control. When 5 appears as the lead number, it shows that control factors are heating up – the SAFent is losing control. His thyroid troubles (anxieties) (10) are causing him to lose control (5).

Q. How does <u>not being able to control</u> relate to have <u>problems with job</u>?

Anchor: For the anchor (22) we use the emotion word listed on the Tamper/SAF Operative Chart, which is anger (parathyroid).

This particular chain sequence shows that certain energies in his system cause him to create the effect of losing control. He is not able to see another's point of view (22) (can't dissect it) and therefore, he is not able to control (5) the situation.

Q. How does <u>anger</u> relate to <u>problems with job</u>?

This is how the chain reads: He is so anxious (10) about his own safety and ability to protect himself (the thyroid is a protection mechanism) that he loses control (5). The anchor holds it all in place: Through his inability to see the other's point of view (22), he worries about his own safety and thus loses control (5).

The trauma for this SAFent was trouble with his job and his worries about losing it. He was not able to accept or implement his boss's ideas, didn't agree with him, and this caused worries about job security. Not acknowledging his anger toward boss caused him to feel out of control and he worried constantly.

After putting this present time scenario all together, SAFent laughed. "This reminds me of a time when I was young and my mom wouldn't let me play with my friends at the creek. I was angry and later went anyway. By myself. As I stepped on a slippery rock, I lost my balance, and in the second before I fell into the water, I envisioned my mother. The whole way home I worried about what I would say."

To further examine this chain, let's look for the up-links and see what we can glean from those. Use the index to locate the up-link explanations.

Sample Chain: <u>5</u>-4-6-<u>10</u>-12-14-<u>22</u>

Up-links:

4-6

"Civilization disease," too many recordings are coming in that can't be digested. This crosses over to physical digestion as well.

6-10

None

10-12

Misunderstood situation. Can't understand new concepts, energy exhaustion. Confusions are present that must be sorted out quickly.

12-14

None

14-22

Angry about situation, but picking the wrong target. Conceptually angry at all the troubles that are befalling him and not coping with any of them.

A third way to examine this trauma chain is by following the stratified history of the emotions it represents, either left to right (present into the past) or by right to left (past time into the present). To do this, you will re-read the sections in chapter 5 that relate to the organs and glands for the numbers in the chain.

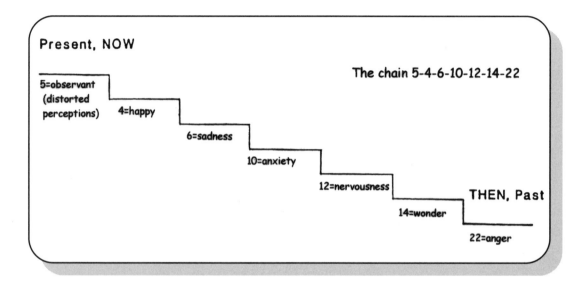

Tamper/SAF Operative Chart

	Condition LEAD	Organ CORE	Emotion ANCHOR
1.	protection	thymus	aggression
2.	synchronize	heart	love
3.	detoxify	colon	hate
4.	digestion	stomach	happy
5.	coordinate	anterior pituitary	observant
6.	transmutation	liver	sadness
7.	vaporization	lungs	monotony
8.	reproduction	sex organs	apathy
9.	locomotion	bones/muscles	pain
10.	metabolization	thyroid	anxiety
11.	circulation	veins/arteries	resentment
12.	electrification	brain	nervousness
13.	capacitance	adrenals	courage
14.	analyzation	mind	wonder
15.	evaluation	senses	attention
16.	filtration	kidneys	fear
17/18.	equalize	endocrine	conservative
19.	demarcation	skin	boredom
20.	location	pancreas	laughter
21.	liquification	posterior pituitary	grief
22.	experience	parathyroid	anger
23.	rejection	spleen	antagonize
24.	acceptance	lymph	enthusiasm

SAF Stress 120 Questionnaire

0 – Never, **1** – Rarely, **2** – Occasionally, **3** – Regularly, **4** – Often, **5** – Very Often

GROUP 1
1. Are you aggressive? _____
2. Do you push yourself too hard? _____
3. Do you usually get your way? _____
4. Are you protective? _____
5. Do you overreact? _____
                                    Total _____

GROUP 2
1. Are you overly sensitive to criticism? _____
2. Do you feel like your heart is broken? _____
3. Do you feel like you are denied love? _____
4. Do you feel that life isn't worth living without your loved one? _____
5. Have you been rejected by someone? _____
                                    Total _____

GROUP 3
1. Do you hold grudges? _____
2. Do you have ongoing feuds with other people? _____
3. Do you blame everyone else for your own problems? _____
4. Do others rub you the wrong way? _____
5. Do you hate your situation? _____
                                    Total _____

GROUP 4
1. Do you have difficulty understanding new information? _____
2. Is it hard to digest situations? _____
3. Do you pretend everything is fine? _____
4. Are you unhappy? _____
5. Does your stomach feel bloated? _____
                                    Total _____

GROUP 5
1. Do you need to get coordinated? _____
2. Do you have to control others? _____
3. Do you feel controlled? _____
4. Do you feel pressure in your chest? _____
5. Do your limbs feel stiff? _____
                                    Total _____

GROUP 6
1. Do you feel depressed? _____
2. Do you feel tired after eating? _____
3. Are you sad? _____
4. Do you feel a constant need for company? _____
5. Do you feel irritated? _____
                                    Total _____

GROUP 7
1. Are you stuck in a rut? _____
2. Are you tired of the same routine? _____
3. Do you need room to breathe? _____
4. Do you feel stifled? _____
5. Do you have suffocation attacks? _____
                                    Total _____

GROUP 8
1. Do you get flushes of heat? _____
2. Do you have cold perspiration? _____
3. Do you feel sexually stimulated? _____
4. Are you apathetic? _____
5. Are you physically weak? _____
                                    Total _____

GROUP 9
1. Do you withhold things that bother you? _____
2. Do you feel overworked? _____
3. Do you refuse to talk about your problems? _____
4. Do temperature changes affect your condition? _____
5. Is someone getting in your way? _____
　　　　　　Total _____

GROUP 10
1. Are you anxious? _____
2. Are you forgetful? _____
3. Do you feel lightheaded or dizzy? _____
4. Do you have a tendency toward fearfulness? _____
5. Do you feel like you can't take the heat? _____
　　　　　　Total _____

GROUP 11
1. Do you feel someone took your place? _____
2. Did someone else get credit for your work? _____
3. Do you deserve something that someone else has? _____
4. Do you resent another's success? _____
5. Do you feel you are never rewarded for what you do? _____
　　　　　　Total _____

GROUP 12
1. Do you jump at the slightest noise? _____
2. Are you nervous? _____
3. Do you have mental conflicts of long duration? _____
4. Are you a light sleeper? _____
5. Do you have projects and plans left undone? _____
　　　　　　Total _____

GROUP 13
1. Are you exhausted? _____
2. Do you feel like you need courage? _____
3. Are you worried? _____
4. Do you feel like people are slowly draining your energy? _____
5. Do you dislike to talk to people about your condition? _____
　　　　　　Total _____

GROUP 14
1. Are you concerned? _____
2. Does the unknown upset you? _____
3. Do you wonder "how you're going to figure this one out?" _____
4. Is your head filled with thoughts? _____
5. Do you sense that something bad might happen? _____
　　　　　　Total _____

GROUP 15
1. Do you feel like you need more energy? _____
2. Do you feel as though you are "getting old"? _____
3. Do you feel worn out? _____
4. Are you sensitive to sun, heat, and other forms of radiation? _____
5. Do you have difficulty concentrating? _____
　　　　　　Total _____

GROUP 16
1. Do you feel like running away? _____
2. Do you have unexplained fears? _____
3. Are you overly concerned about what you eat? _____
4. Are you shy? _____
5. Are you nauseated when under pressure? _____
　　　　　　Total _____

GROUP 17/18

1. Do you feel chilly? _____
2. Do you have high blood pressure? _____
3. Does it hurt to think? _____
4. Do you have a bad memory? _____
5. Do you have to get up to go to the bathroom in the middle of the night? _____
6. Are you unstable? _____
7. Has your behavior changed? (You do not act like yourself) _____
8. Do you feel a constant need for something to eat? _____
9. Is your balance poor? _____
10. Do you have sexual disturbances? (Impotence, frigidity, etc.) _____

Total _____

Adjusted Total _____

GROUP 19

1. Are you bored? _____
2. Are you tired of the same situations? _____
3. Have you lost the ability to set priorities? _____
4. Is it hard to distinguish one situation from another? _____
5. Do you tremble all over? _____

Total _____

GROUP 20

1. Are you under a lot of stress? _____
2. Do you feel that you have low stamina? _____
3. Do you feel that you have some hidden condition? _____
4. Do you find it difficult to laugh off your troubles? _____
5. Do you have odd facial expressions? _____

Total _____

GROUP 21

1. Have you lost a loved one? _____
2. Have you lost a job/position? _____
3. Do you feel you will lose at most anything you try? _____
4. Do you feel nervous tension after a minimal amount of physical activity? _____
5. Do your palms sweat? _____

Total _____

GROUP 22

1. Do you have a bad temper? _____
2. Are you impatient? _____
3. Do you find fault easily? _____
4. Do you curse and swear? _____
5. Are you angry about your situation? _____

Total _____

GROUP 23

1. Do you reject others? _____
2. Do you feel as though you need to inhale fresh air? _____
3. Have you had a shock or a trauma? _____
4. Are you antagonized by others? _____
5. Is your breathing irregular? _____

Total _____

GROUP 24

1. Are you addicted to drugs (especially narcotics?) _____
2. Do you drink alcohol? _____
3. Do you smoke cigarettes, pipes, cigars, or chew tobacco? _____
4. Are you easily excitable? _____
5. Are you easily prone to sighing and sobbing? _____

Total _____

No directions are given in this book for the Questionnaire. The CD-ROM contains the questions and once you've answered them, it will automatically give you your chain and lead, core and anchor numbers.

Index

must be free flowing, 33
of the trauma, 53
enthusiasm, 189
entity changes form, 45
equalize, 151
evaluation, 128
experience, 179

F

failure, 145, 146
fear, 137
filtration, 138

G

Galileo, 9, 71
genesis, 38
genetic blueprint, 194
  changeover, 187
  code, 36
  history and disease, 47
  mental image banks, 49
  research, 193-194
  timetable, 37
goal of SAF, 29
grid work of disease, 67
grid work of the sun, 67
grief, 173

H

happy, 84
harmony, 52
hate, 81
heart, 78-80
  emotion, 78
  condition, 79
  mental aspects, 80
  physical aspects, 80
hemophilia, 194
Hiroshima, 69

homeopathic remedies, 120, 121
homesick, 169
homosexuality, 150-151
hormone imbalance, 150
human being, what is, 17
human beings think in sequences, 85
hypnosis, 129
hypothalamus, 126-136
  condition, 128
  emotion, 127
  mental aspects, 129
  physical aspects, 133

I

ice cream incident, 20, 23, 49, 50
immortality, 179
immunity, 10, 12
  on any level, 51
indigestion, mental and spiritual, 60
  confusion, 60
infiltration, loss of energy, 53
infrared
  detector, 45
  face template, 163
  sensitizer, 156
  image, 3D, 163
interference detectors, 42

J

Joseph R. Scogna, Jr., 5, 10, 69, 164

K

kidneys and bladder, 137-148
  condition, 138
  emotion, 137
  mental aspects, 142
  physical aspects, 147

Numbers and Combinations

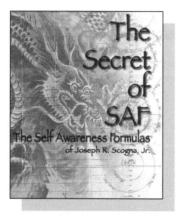
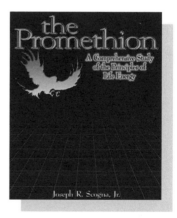

End-User License Agreement

READ THIS: You should carefully read these terms and conditions before opening the software packet included with SAF Simplified-Self Awareness Formulas ("Book"). This is a license agreement ("Agreement") between you and Kathy M. Scogna ("Copyright Owner"). By breaking the seal on the accompanying CD you acknowledge that you have read and accept the terms and conditions of the End-User License Agreement. If you do not agree and do not want to be bound by such terms and conditions, promptly return the Book and unopened software packet to the place you obtained them for a full refund.

1. **License Grant.** Kathy M. Scogna (Copyright Owner) grants to you a nonexclusive license to use one copy of the enclosed software program solely for your own personal purposes on a single computer. Copyright Owner reserves all proprietary rights and ownership.

2. **Ownership.** Kathy M. Scogna is the owner of all right, title, and interest, including copyright, in and to the compilation of the Software recorded on the CD-ROM ("Software Media").

3. **Restrictions on Use and Transfer.** You may not (i) rent or lease the Software or Software Media, (ii) copy or reproduce through a network system, subscriber program or bulletin-board system or (iii) modify, adapt or create derivative works based on the Software. (iv) You may not reverse engineer, decompile or disassemble the Software.

4. **Limited Warranty.** (i) Copyright Owner warrants that the Software and Software Media are free from defects in materials and workmanship under normal use for a period of sixty (60) days from the date of purchase of the Book. If Copyright Owner receives notification within the warranty period of defects in materials or workmanship, Copyright Owner will replace the defective Software Media. (ii) Copyright Owner disclaims all other warranties, express or implied, including without limitation implied warranties of merchantability and fitness for a particular purpose, with respect to the software, the program, the source code contained, and the techniques described in this Book. Copyright Owner does not warrant that the functions contained in the software will meet your requirements or that the operation will be error free.

5. **Remedies.** Copyright Owner's entire liability and your exclusive remedy for defects in materials and workmanship shall be limited to replacement of the Software Media, which must be returned along with the Book to Life Energy Publications with a copy of your receipt at the following address: Life Energy Publications, 695 N. Church Road, Wernersville, Pennsylvania, 19565. This Limited Warranty is void if failure of the Software Media has resulted from accident, abuse, or misapplication. Any replacement Software Media/Book will be warranted for the remainder of the original warranty period or thirty (30) days, whichever is longer. In no event shall Copyright Owner be liable for any damages whatsoever arising from the use or inability to use the Book or the Software.

6. **General.** This agreement shall be governed by and construed in accordance with the laws of the Commonwealth of Pennsylvania (without regard to conflicts of law principles), except as to matters pertaining to Federal copyright laws which shall be governed by the laws of the United States of America. This agreement shall be treated as though it were executed and performed in, and any cause of action with respect to the Book and/or Software must be brought solely in Pennsylvania. All actions must be subject to the limitations set forth in this Agreement.

7. This agreement constitutes the entire understanding and agreement of the parties and revokes and supercedes all prior or contemporaneous agreements, oral or written. If any one or more provisions contained in this Agreement are held by any court or tribunal to be invalid, illegal, or otherwise unenforceable, each and every other provision shall remain in full force and effect.